Why Are You Sick?

How to reclaim your health with the Ultimate Health Model™

Benjamin L. Smith

Disclaimer: I am not a medical professional. I am not providing healthcare, medical, or nutritional therapy services or attempting to diagnose, treat, prevent, or cure any physical, mental, or emotional issue. The information in my book is for informational purposes only and is not intended to substitute professional medical advice, diagnoses, or treatment. Always seek advice from your physician or other qualified healthcare provider before undertaking a new health regimen. Do not disregard medical advice or delay seeking medical advice because of the information you read in this book. Do not start or stop any medications without speaking to your medical or mental health provider.

Visit www.ultimatehealthmodel.com for resources in your quest for health.

Copyright © 2024 Benjamin Smith

All Rights Reserved.

No content of this book may be copied, excerpted, replicated, or shared without the permission of the author.

Published by SuburbanBuzz.com LLC

ISBN: 978-1-959446-33-0

DEDICATION

This book is dedicated to those I have lost to cancer and the millions of people who seek a better, healthier way to live. Thank you for sharing my message.

CONTENTS

ACKNOWLEDGMENTS i
FOREWORD By Tim Smith iii
INTRODUCTION The Lies We're Told 1
CHAPTER 1 A World of Myths 7
CHAPTER 2 The Ultimate Health Model™ 17
CHAPTER 3 Body Design 45
CHAPTER 4 Breathing 73
CHAPTER 5 Sleeping 95
CHAPTER 6 Structured Water 115
CHAPTER 7 Food 143
CHAPTER 8 Movement 183
CHAPTER 9 Environment 203
CHAPTER 10 Thoughts and Feelings 223
CHAPTER 11 What If? 235
ABOUT THE AUTHOR 241

ACKNOWLEDGMENTS

I thank everyone who inspired and shaped this book. From my own health journey to copious digging and research, I appreciate the many friends and mentors who were instrumental along the way. You know who you are and what you mean to this project.

FOREWORD
The Ultimate Health Model™
By Tim Smith

If you get confused by all the thousands of health books out there and aren't sure which one to believe, you aren't alone. There are so many experts—each with his or her own formula for achieving perfect health. Most of them advocate for a single approach. They imply if you just adopt this exercise regimen or this diet or this supplement or avoid these foods, etc., then you will lose weight, feel better, have more energy, improve your endurance, sleep better… you know the story.

But how does following one of these magic bullet approaches actually work overtime? Did you keep the weight off? Did your arthritis improve? Did your allergies get better? Are you getting more sleep, have more energy, fewer headaches, better focus, etc.?

I'm not a health expert. I'm just a guy who was introduced to the Ultimate Health Model™ in the spring of 2023. Some parts of the model resonated with what I already knew, some was new, and some was beyond my understanding. But the common sense, logic and science behind this approach convinced me to begin trying some of what Ben Smith (no relation) writes about in this book.

Over a few weeks, my arthritis nearly disappeared.

My energy level continued to rise, and I noticed myself losing weight for the first time in years—WITHOUT DIETING! My overall sense of wellness is significantly higher than before I started implementing the recommendations in his book.

But that's the beauty of his wellness "model." Dig in where you are and start focusing on a few changes. Learn about the lifestyle factors. Start increasing the healthy ones and reducing or eliminating the unhealthy ones. Whether it's less sugar and carbs, better water, more movement, meditation—whatever—get started with some of it. The more you do, the more results you will experience.

This short, easy-to-read book offers a great blend of common sense and surprisingly simple stuff you didn't know that matters. It's a disruptive approach that dispels many of the myths behind health that we take for granted. It also explains why there is so much contradictory information out there. Smith asserts that we are chronically dehydrated—not because we don't drink fluids, but because we do a variety of things that interfere with our body's ability to function as designed. This dehydration, in turn, leads to inflammation that stresses our body and causes discomfort and, ultimately, disease.

The beauty of the Ultimate Health Model™ is that it's an overall approach—not a singular silver bullet that ignores the rest of the important factors behind your health. This is a book that's written for average folks like us. It's easy to read, often humorous, and backed by science that Smith explains in language we can understand. Think of the Ultimate Health Model™ as a road map to plot your way back to optimal health. Our bodies were designed to function optimally, and all we need to do is learn how to connect the right dots.

INTRODUCTION
The Lies We're Told

Life is to be enjoyed, not simply endured.

~ Willard Gaylin

Does it sometimes feel like reclaiming our health is just out of reach?

Do you feel like you're working hard just to get through the day, surviving instead of thriving? Are you stressed out? Do you feel that your vitality is gone? Maybe when you were twenty, everything was great, but at thirty, or forty, or fifty, you feel like it's all downhill from here. Your body's not working as well as when you were a kid. Everything aches, and everyone says that the older you get, the worse it will be.

That's why I'm sharing the Ultimate Health Model™.

Have you been following mainstream advice but not getting better? You might have type 2 diabetes, heart disease, high blood pressure, allergies, migraines, bad breath, acid reflux, or a myriad of other health ailments. Maybe you suffer from headaches or feel sluggish when you should have energy. You might even have dementia, Alzheimer's, or cancer.

Doctors treat your symptoms but not the underlying root causes. You're still sick, and you don't know why.

Or maybe you're unhappy with your weight. You try to diet, but every time you drop a pound, you gain it right back. You can't lose those stubborn inches no matter how much you try. You have a beer belly or pregnancy weight you can't lose. Your hormones are out of balance, and you're constantly pressured by society's messages into thinking this is *all your fault*.

You're told to exercise more and eat less. How's that workin' for ya? If I hear that trite and obviously incorrect mantra one more time, I'm going to puke!

This leaves you feeling discouraged and disappointed. You're becoming resigned to a life of pain. You can't help but wonder . . . *If all these treatments are supposed to work, and all the mainstream health knowledge is right, why is everyone still sick?* You feel like you've followed the rainbow but found no pot of gold. Just misery.

It doesn't have to be this way. All of that can change, and there *is* a way to get that pot of gold. Health and vitality *are* waiting for you. Why are you sick? It isn't your fault. You've just had the wool pulled over your eyes and been sent down the wrong road.

It's time to open your eyes to the truth.

Reclaim Your Health

What if I told you I had the proverbial key to unlocking your health challenges? Would you proclaim, "Hallelujah?"

I've been researching health practices for fifteen years to find the truth the world doesn't acknowledge. I've learned just how much we know but don't talk about when it comes to our overall health and wellness. I've distilled the unconventional answers I discovered into the Ultimate Health Model™, founded on a symbiotic relationship between underlying cellular factors and causative factors that determine your health status.

In this book, you will see the myths you've been told and how those lies, stripped away, reveal the truth. At the end of the day, you'll be able to put your questions into visual form through my Ultimate Health Model™.

If you're looking for a typical self-help book, this isn't for you. If you want a secret formula or fad diet for what to eat and how to lose weight, this isn't for you. Psst...there is no secret formula! Eat one ingredient, whole food! Something your great-grandma would recognize!

Do you want to know *why* you're overweight? Do you want to know what causes inflammation and how to fight it? Do you want to know the truths about your health that no one talks about? Do you want to know why you're sick and how to get better?

Then you're in the right place.

I'm not going to sugarcoat this for you. This book will get raw and down to the "nitty-gritty." I might use profanity and be in your face, but this is the slap you need to wake up! This is your life we are talking about—and the quality of it, for that matter.

This book gets you to the root causes of the health conditions that are impacting your life and teaches you how to treat them. It shares ideas that no one else has put together in one resource guide. This is fascinating, potentially life-changing information that you've possibly never known until now.

If you follow the practices and systems in this book, you'll have better health. Your body will be more in balance. You'll experience more vitality, energy, and excitement about life. You will understand that your poor health isn't your fault.

It might take a month. It might take six months. But I guarantee you that you will start to feel better. You will have more hope for your health, and you'll see the light, maybe for the first time in a long time.

A Future of Vitality

I know what these principles can do because I've put them all into practice in my own life. I've seen the benefits firsthand. I'm a certified health coach, and I practice what I preach.

I'm not a doctor. I'm not a scientist, a dietician, or a nutritionist. Frankly, I didn't want to train in any of those disciplines. Most mainstream doctors do very little investigation despite a world of dubious health outcomes. Those "experts" are taught to think a certain way, and that's not me. They don't ask the "whys"—they just regurgitate information, regardless of whether that information is questionable. WTF?

So if you're looking at the claims above and wondering, *Who is this guy? What does he think he knows?* The answer is simple: I'm someone who's been paying attention. I voraciously read everything I can get my hands on. I do the research, speak with experts in their respective fields, and then come to my own conclusions. I test my hypotheses by putting them into practice in my own life. And when I see the results, I share my findings with those around me.

I'm not infallible. I feel compelled to publish this book as I observe the world around me, and believe I might have some answers. I have done my best to share largely unexplored, complex topics. I've also compiled what's already out there and some new information that I've studied and theorized. If it makes sense, use it. If it doesn't, ignore it. If a fact is out of place, please bring it to my attention on my website at ultimatehealthmodel.com.

But on the whole, I believe the book is founded on correct information. It's an exercise in free will, and I'm a living example of doing just that. I truly believe in the Ultimate Health Model™ and can't wait to see its impact on your health and vitality. You're going to look better, feel better, and have hope for the future—for your health and your independence. I have confidence that even if things in your life have gotten really bad, they will improve if you follow these health practices.

The universe wants you to be healthy. Once you understand that and how to think outside the box, you will have health and vitality. The puzzle pieces of your health are all there. Open your mind to the goodness around you, and you will finally be able to see the big picture of your health.

Are you ready? It's time to start your health and wellness boot camp!

CHAPTER 1
A World of Myths

It is estimated that 12 million children suffer from asthma, and several thousand die every year. Let us declare an end to asthma in less than five years. Let us save children from the constant fear of suffocation because they do not recognize they are thirsty for water.
~ Dr. Batmanghelidj, author of Your Body's Many Cries for Water

The quote above is very personal to me. I had childhood asthma, and it almost killed me a few times. To anyone who has asthma, I know your pain, anxiety, and struggles. The contributing causes are due to the factors in my health model, and this both pisses me off and gives me hope to help other's suffering.

I breathed through my mouth rather than my nose, not knowing it was causing dehydration. I believe dehydration causes an allergic reaction due to the loss of water. I believe structured water is an antihistamine, yet no doctor shared this information with me. We will discuss the fascinating properties of water in later chapters.

I know what it's like to be hungry all the time, yet never satisfied. I know what it's like to have allergies, hay fever, and acid reflux. I know the challenges you're going through.

And I know that it's not your fault.

Chronic Disease Is Everywhere

No, it's not your fault you're sick. It's not your fault you're tired. We live in a world of myths, falsehoods, and overwhelming ignorance about the fundamental pillars of health. Nutritional studies are seriously flawed to the point of becoming completely useless for determining causation. When they say a study is statistically powerful because X number of people participated, that really doesn't matter IF the study is flawed.

It's important to mention how these studies are done. Some are called "observational" studies. Researchers give participants questionnaires and ask them what they ate over a given period of time. How accurate do you think that could possibly be? Sorting through the facts and fiction takes decades; believe me, I know.

If you learn nothing else from this book, remember that *causation* is not *association*. I know it's difficult to go against the establishment, mainstream media, and what has been forced down our proverbial throats for decades, but it's worth a shot if you might feel better, isn't it?

Consider the quotes below:

> *Today, an estimated 133 million Americans – nearly half the population – suffer from at least one chronic illness, such as hypertension, heart disease and arthritis …*
> ~ American Hospital Association

> *Each year approximately 30.4 million deaths worldwide are the result of chronic disease.*
> ~ American Institute for Cancer Research

The good news is that you feel the way you do for a reason. There's a monster at the heart of the maze, which I call "chronic cellular oxidative stress." Cellular oxidative stress is a threat to the cells. Think of it this way: the cells are scared because their survival is endangered. If they could speak, they'd say, "Dude, keep these threats away from me!" What are the threats? I explain them in the Ultimate Health

Model™ coming up in Chapter 2.

This chronic cellular stress is what's spinning in the background, along with the other symbiotic cellular factors—like chronic dehydration and inflammation, dysfunctional mitochondria, and a suppressed immune system. All are contributing to your health challenges.

Before we go any further, let's define a few terms.

- **Acute** means severe and sudden onset not lasting in duration.
- **Chronic** means "long-lasting or reoccurring."
- **Oxidative stress** is the imbalance between damaging molecules in cells (oxidants) and helpful molecules (antioxidants).
- **Inflammation** is "swelling, redness or tenderness of an area especially from injury or infection." Head scratcher: do you think inflammation is different on the inside than the outside? Likely not.
- **Mitochondria**, as we'll see on the model, are the energy-generating part of the cell. This organelle (structure inside the cell) lets the cell do work.

I believe that when you *chronically* activate the circles on the red side of the Ultimate Health Model™, it impacts everything, from making you age more quickly to increasing your risk of diseases like arthritis and cancer. The difference between "chronic" and "acute" is an important distinction I will elaborate on throughout the book.

Think of chronic inflammation like a wound that never completely and properly heals. If you cut yourself, the wound scabs over, then slowly heals from within. But if you pull that scab off, your body must start the healing process all over again. Chronic inflammation is like that wound. Your body keeps scabbing it over, trying to heal. But as long as you're still bombarding your body with new negative factors, the wound will never close.

That's what's going on in your body right now. **Its natural systems of repair are being outpaced by damage, and your body just can't keep up.** Think for a moment of your blood vessels with this scarring analogy. This is *exactly* what happens. The scarring is like the calcium stabilizing the plaque (damage to the artery wall) so they don't burst and possibly put you six feet under. Lightbulb moment!

To embrace better health and give your body what it needs to heal, you need to do everything in your power to reduce the negative lifestyle factors you subject it to and increase the positive ones. Looking at the Ultimate Health Model™ described below in Chapter 2, you want to get off the red chronic disease side and onto the green optimal health side, where all the lifestyle factors are leading, instead, to better health.

Some contributing factors of chronic disease are out of your control. Take, for instance, electromagnetic frequencies (EMFs). They're all around us, and they likely cause chronic inflammation. Unless you hide in a cave in the wilderness somewhere, EMFs are a fact of life. That's why controlling the red chronic disease factors you can regulate is so important.

I've come up with an easy way to know if something is good or bad for you. But first, let me share a personal story.

Family Loss

In 2012, I lost my sister to cancer.

After she died, I was confused, hurt, and bewildered. I wanted to understand why she died and why modern medicine, with all its marvels, hadn't been able to save her. I was so angry. Why didn't the doctors mention **chronic dehydration** as one of the main contributing factors to cancer? How did they not know this?

I started reading about cancer and health. I explored topics that weren't heavily researched. I investigated the design of the human body and the logical conclusions no one was drawing from what we already knew. I began to understand the missing pieces and the puzzle that the information formed. I told myself that it doesn't make sense that someone just gets cancer. Like it was bad luck. Knowing what I knew about the body and how miraculous it was, this did not make sense.

Interesting side note: everyone has cancerous cells, but if your immune system is healthy, it removes them.

I implemented the model I created in my own life, and the change was staggering. For the first time, I had real health and vitality. My inflammation went down, and I lost weight. I had more energy, and I felt younger. Everyone commented on how much healthier and happier I seemed.

Then, a few years after we lost my sister, my mother's cancer returned. She was initially diagnosed in 1985. In the decades since then, her body had been trying to stay healthy despite her contributing to the negative factors in our model.

As scary as it was, I knew that I wasn't helpless this time. I wanted to tell my mom to **avoid sugar** to keep her inflammation down. How was her body going to fight cancer if she suppressed her immune system?

I knew she wouldn't listen to me. I'm not a doctor. I knew my advice would fall on deaf ears.

And in 2019, I lost her.

I was heartbroken. I asked myself, Why do people

do this? Why can't we get out of our heads, away from what we're told, and think about it logically?

I wanted to throw my hands up. If no one would listen, what could I do? A few years later, my brother-in-law's sister was diagnosed with liver cancer, and I watched it happen all over again. That was the trigger that shook me out of my lethargy. The people I loved were sick. I had friends on dialysis and family taking blood pressure medicine. There had to be a better way. I had a message worth sharing—a message that could literally save people's lives.

I researched existing health books and was both thrilled and alarmed to see that no one else was talking about the factors in my model. There was no integrative approach explaining the dynamic relationship between them. Articles were out there, but no one had distilled that knowledge into a book.

So I did. I dug, read, and distilled everything I found into the Ultimate Health Model™. I combined that research with lengthy discussions with experts in these fields to corroborate my hypothesis and challenge my claims.

Thus, I had the answers, but my message wasn't working. I needed to find a medium to share life-saving information with everyone in a way that resonated and compelled the sick to action. The first question you might be asking is why I didn't go to medical school. That way, people would listen to what I say. The answer is in the complexity of my model. They don't teach any of that! Zero! That's why I chose another route.

The first thing I did was to become a certified health coach. I found an organization I trusted, one that shared my philosophy about how to prevent chronic disease and achieve health and well-being. The courses at Primal Health Coaching were fantastic, and I loved my training and certification process. After I graduated, I decided not to take individual coaching clients. I wanted to share my message in a broader way.

"Why don't you write a book?" my friend asked.

It was a lightning bolt. With a book, I could lay out all of the information I had gathered over the years. I could share my message in a way that had never been possible before. I'm so excited to share it all with you. Maybe my work can help shortcut the confusion that I faced. I want you to feel happy, vibrant and energized about your body and health.

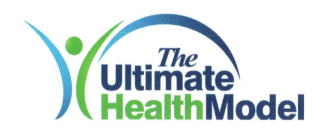

CHAPTER 2
The Ultimate Health Model™

It is health that is the real wealth, and not pieces of gold and silver.
~ Mahatma Gandhi

Get your yellow markers ready. You are in for the educational journey of your life!

What exactly is the Ultimate Health Model™? And how can you apply it in your daily life?

Well, the Ultimate Health Model™ is unlike anything you have seen. Some of it may be familiar, and some of it is likely new to you. Why this model is so unique and important is that it integrates all of the core factors that contribute to health or disease and why. It distills scientific research, health principles and practices, and personal experience over the last decade. It's meant to boost your critical thinking skills and empower you.

Everything I share on these pages is based on research I've found or done. But you're welcome to do your own online research. In fact, I encourage you to find resources, so you can discover what works for you. Of course, you will find a lot of conflicting material out there, but this model is based on what I found to be the most effective practices based on years of trial and error.

I was so passionate about health that I became a health coach. I'm so zealous that my energy sometimes spills onto the page with conversational language and even swear words. Forgive me in advance. I want to break through the veil of "expertise" we've all been fed and share my enthusiasm.

There's an answer in these pages for any question and objection you have. When you have the foundational knowledge you need, the Ultimate Health Model™ becomes your solution. **Nothing else is stopping you but you.**

You'll walk away with a different understanding of why you feel the way you do. You'll be able to put the puzzle pieces together and see the bigger picture—a better life, waiting just at the bend in the road.

That all starts with a deeper understanding of how the systems and processes in your body work.

Your Guide to Better Health

After years of pulling together information from hundreds of different sources, I designed a model for ultimate health. I integrated and synthesized available information and came up with a formula that is beautiful in its simplicity. There is a green side (positive) and a red side (negative), and you can ask it any questions you want. The answers will always be the same. You'll see so in the graphic.

The premise of my health model is simple: the human body is perfect. It's been around as a species for approximately four million years. The body and the universe are one and the same. There's nothing out of place. If an organ system in the body isn't functioning at optimal capacity, there has to be a reason. No, your type 2 diabetes isn't a punishment. Your body is not trying to hurt you. It's simply trying to protect itself. Likewise, there is a reason for your varicose veins, your heart murmur, or any affliction you've experienced.

The Ultimate Health Model™ charts the factors that lead to chronic disease (including lifestyle factors) versus the factors that lead to optimal health. The most important lifestyle areas and factors are **breath, sleep, water, food, movement, environment, and thoughts and emotions**. They're not all-encompassing, but they are absolutely the foundation of everything that impacts the five circles you'll see in the Ultimate Health Model™ below.

You'll see the interrelationship between the cellular and lifestyle factors that positively and negatively impact our health. These cellular factors are what is happening in the body behind the scenes.

If you truly understand the Ultimate Health Model™, you'll understand what's going on in your body at a cellular level. The power of this model is that it lets you control your health. By understanding which factors contribute to poor health, you don't have to rely on anyone else's opinions to know what's good for your body.

Below is a visual guide and quick summary so you can see exactly how to use The Ultimate Health Model™ and diagnose your own health problems—just like I did for myself. You might ask, "Why are there cartoon characters? This doesn't look like your typical health book." I'm trying to explain about your health in a whole different way. I chose to use cartoons as a way to help describe the concepts more clearly and make them more engaging and identifiable. I hope you find it useful. My heartfelt desire is to help you and the ones you love lead happier, healthier, and longer lives.

Allow me to now introduce Healthy Heidi & Hank and Diseased Debbie & Dan.

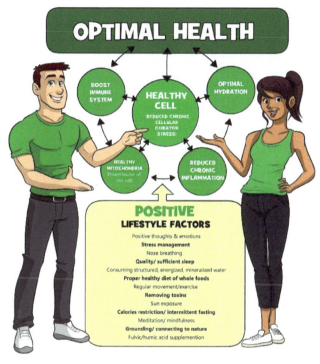
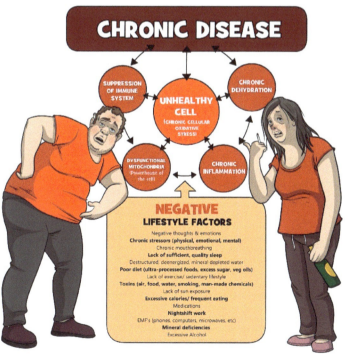

Healthy Cells Vs. Unhealthy Cells

Over the last decade, I've constantly asked myself questions. I wanted to get to the root cause of the things I was reading about in my studies. **I knew the universe was perfect, and the body would not "do something" for no reason.** I asked why things happened. What caused them? Where does disease and illness come from?

Inspired by new topics, I would read up on a new area, combine it with the information that already existed, and apply it to what I knew in order to form new conclusions. "Why" drove my life for many years.

Those years of study, of bridging connections between existing modalities, led me to develop my own model for optimal health. Everytime I found a new answer to one of my whys, I plugged it into the diagram and saw that it had a place there. Soon, I had the complete model, laying out the five circles on the wheels of positive and negative health and the lifestyle factors that create movement on the Ultimate Health Model™.

Understanding this model will help you change your health altogether. Armed with a concrete understanding of your own health, you are empowered to do a 180 in your behaviors. You will understand how the circles relate and how to change your health by changing your lifestyle factors—all by learning the ins and outs of the Ultimate Health Model™.

This model is the foundation of this book. It creates a visual perspective on how the five circles interrelate. On the side of Optimal Health, the five positive circles impact our health in positive ways. On the opposite side of Chronic Disease, the five negative circles impact our health in negative ways.

On each side, all five circles are linked, including the middle circles on their respective sides. You can see the relationship between the circles, the lifestyle factors, and the overarching pinnacles at the top: chronic disease or optimal health. That is why the arrows are omnidirectional.

Now let me explain the conditions in the five sets of circles. What do we do that helps us, and what do we do that hurts us? I added lifestyle factors to take the guesswork out of controlling your health. If you want to optimize your health, all you have to do is choose green lifestyle factors. If you feel sick and you want to know why, look at the list of red lifestyle factors and see how many of them you engage in. The math is simple. This also explains what the book cover is about. "Green side good, red side bad" is our slogan. Make sense now?

Observe the Circles

Why are the circles for unhealthy/healthy cells larger on the model, you might ask? Well, you'll see why when you take a closer look. All the circles either create healthy or unhealthy cells because of their interdependent relationships.

- **Healthy / Unhealthy cells:** I'm leading with healthy/unhealthy cells because it's the most important circle on the model. All these processes in the circles end up with a healthy or unhealthy cell and either high or low oxidative stress. Cellular oxidative stress is when the antioxidant systems of the cell are overwhelmed by the prooxidant factors. The definition of the term oxidation is the oxygen reacting with a substance and causing the displacement of electrons. When out of balance, this is bad. The prooxidant, or "oxidation" factors are the red lifestyle factors, and the antioxidant factors are on the green side. Blueberries aren't your savior. Supposed "antioxidant" juice drinks won't save you either. It's more than that. Grounding is an antioxidant. Structured water is an antioxidant. Nose breathing with your mouth closed is an antioxidant! More about all of this later.

- **Optimal hydration / Chronic dehydration:** Hydration is critical for optimal bodily functioning. I cannot stress this enough. As little as a two percent hydration deficit can cause symptoms like migraine headaches, joint pain, or virtually anything. How does this relate to the rest of the circles? People are dehydrated and don't even know it. I believe chronic dehydration is the most important circle on the model. It activates all other circles, simple as that. As we will discuss, all the red lifestyle factors are causing this problem, and that's why seventy-five percent or more of the population could be in trouble.

- **Boosted immune system / Suppression of the immune system:** Your immune system keeps your body healthy. The immune system contains two parts: innate and adaptive. Think of the immune system like the armed forces. You've got soldiers, generals, lieutenants, even suicide bombers. The analogies that can be drawn are fascinating. Understand that "suppression of the immune system" means it's being chronically overactivated. This overactivation weakens it over time. The body can actually turn it off and shut it down due to fatigue. It has to balance itself in some way. And as discussed in the next bullet point, the immune system comes to the aid when there is inflammation, which can be chronic or acute. We will cover how this all occurs—and how your immune system may be impacted—in more detail in later chapters.

- **Reduced chronic inflammation / Chronic inflammation:** Inflammation is mainly the result of chronic dehydration and stress on the cells. It's the wound that never heals unless you follow the points on the green side. This is all related but extremely complex and simple at the same time. Interesting side note: people say when you get older, your metabolism slows down. "I can't lose the belly because I'm getting older." Wrong! It's because your inflammation has become chronic. The more inflammation, the more you gain weight or are unable to lose weight.

- **Healthy mitochondria / Dysfunctional mitochondria:** Mitochondria are probably the most important organelles (a specialized part of a cell that has an assigned function). Why? In addition to producing much of the energy for the cell, mitochondria control many other aspects of cell life, like whether a cell lives, dies, or proliferates. Chronic dehydration causes massive mitochondrial dysfunction. You can see how dysfunction of this remarkable part of the cell can contribute to chronic disease.

The wheels of health are drawn in a circuit. Each one has two arrows, one leading to the factor below and one to the factor above. That can be misleading. The truth is that all of the circles on the model are interconnected on their perspective sides. Chronic dehydration can lead to chronic inflammation can lead to suppression of the immune system can lead to mitochondrial dysfunction—the four horsemen of the bodily apocalypse. On the green side, you have four unicorns that create magic—boost to the immune system, optimal hydration, healthy mitochondria, and reduced chronic inflammation. They feed into each other seamlessly, creating a network of health impacts that all lead to chronic disease or optimum health. They describe exactly what's happening to you at all times, all day, every day, for your whole life. They leave nothing out.

And when I say chronic disease, I don't just mean cancer and type 2 diabetes. We often ignore other conditions like acid reflux, gout, arthritis, and fibromyalgia, which are all inflammatory processes. As the model states, any and ALL chronic conditions, from psoriasis to shingles to a fever to a nosebleed, are all inflammatory-based. They all lead to oxidative stress on the cells, which in turn creates an "unhealthy cell."

You may be wondering, *What about genetics? Don't I have a predisposition to certain diseases?* A component of genetics is involved, but it's much smaller than you likely believe. Cancer and type 2 diabetes have a genetic element, but they're impacted by epigenetics, a process in which your lifestyle factors impact and change how your genes are expressed. You'll learn more about these lifestyle factors later, and you'll see how they interact with the circles. **Essentially, the environment is controlling your genes, not your** fate.

This brings me to another lie about genetics that we've been told, and it really pisses me off. The mainstream says that male pattern baldness and hair loss or androgenic alopecia is controlled by genes, and these are the shitty cards you're dealt in life. The truth is this is mostly an autoimmune condition brought on and exacerbated by the red lifestyle factors. I suffered from this myself, and I know the pain, anxiety, and self-consciousness it brings. My f'ckn mouth breathing and massive carb addiction were contributing to this and causing me to look like a fuzzy cue ball. Yep! If you want to keep your flowing locks into your golden years, embrace the green lifestyle factors!

Some lifestyle factors are so big—like nose breathing vs. mouth breathing—that they take up an entire chapter. Others can be encompassed as subpoints in another topic. You'll learn about night-shift workers, for instance, in the Sleep Chapter. All of these lifestyle factors tie back into the positive and negative circles of the Ultimate Health Model™.

Let's look at each of the lifestyle factors that impact your health. Understand that each factor impacts all circles in the wheel simultaneously to different degrees. This is intended to give you an overview of your learning.

Lifestyle Factors

Now that you understand the red and green circles, we can break down the lifestyle factors. Think of the Ultimate Health Model™ as a roadmap to get you healthy at any age. On the bright side, the positive lifestyle changes you make now will help you build long-lasting optimal health. Below, you'll see a comparison of negative factors and the benefits of moving to the green side and tweaking your lifestyle.

✓ **Positive Thoughts / Emotions:** Positive thoughts and emotions reduce stress on the cells and the body itself. Reduced stress means improved digestion, improved cardiovascular system, reduced inflammation, increased hydration, and improved immune function. It facilitates all cellular functions to work properly. This is exactly what the circles tell you on the green side. Also, do you ever wonder if water holds consciousness? I believe so. Positive thoughts and emotions help structure your body's water, and guess what? Structured water is one of the green lifestyle factors. Sounds far out there or is this starting to sink in? Just wait until you read the chapter on water. You'll learn all about water's long memory.

✗ **Negative Thoughts / Emotions:** We all know that negative thoughts can contribute to the progression of disease. Why? Because they cause cellular stress and all the other circles to engage.

✅ **Stress Management (Physical, Emotional, Mental):** When you're stressed, you activate the sympathetic nervous system. You enter flight-or-fight mode, and all of your healing functions cease. When you can control that stress, you are able to use your parasympathetic nervous system and enter the rest-and-digest phase, where your body heals. It's that simple.

❌ **Chronic Stressors:** Maybe you're stressed out because you lost your job, your husband left you, someone in your family died, or you have a chronic disease. This stress, even though it's not life-threatening, makes your body react like it's metaphorically trying to escape from a saber-tooth tiger. That triggers your body to go into a host of chemical and biological reactions. One of these hormones is cortisol, and you've probably heard how stress increases this hormone. Interestingly, most people think cortisol is the boogyman, but it actually has an important job to do, like everything in the body. Cortisol is actually an anti-inflammatory and an immune system enhancer when it's not chronically activated. Take part in minimizing your stress to "rest and digest" effectively.

***

✅ **Nose Breathing:** When you breathe through your nose, you take in more oxygen. We'll discuss how this really works in the Breathing Chapter.

❌ **Chronic Mouth Breathing:** Breathing through your mouth brings in less oxygen than breathing through your nose. This probably sounds counterintuitive, but it will be explained in later chapters. Mouth breathing hurts your health long term and activates *all* the circles on the red side.

***

✅ **Sufficient Sleep:** Your body runs on circadian rhythms and a biological clock. When you have quality, sufficient sleep, your body is able to enter the repair-and-restore cycle (with the help of melatonin, a major antioxidant). A majority of the melatonin is produced inside the mitochondria of cells instead of the pineal gland in the brain. For those who participate in night shift work, your circadian rhythm is affected, and your body produces the most melatonin when you are resting in the dark. So when you're up at night, your "internal housekeeping" is affected. Fortunately for the people keeping the nights hummin' and the beer a flowin', the melatonin synthesized in the mitochondria is less circadian-dependent. If you have to do night shift work, try to do as many things on the green side as possible.

✗ **Lack of Quality Sleep:** For the same reasons that night-shift work hurts your body, not getting enough sleep is harmful. Lack of sleep creates massive stress on the cells because they can't be repaired sufficiently. And then, guess what happens? The Wheel of Doom on the red side spins round and round. For example, we are evolutionarily designed to digest food in the daytime and sleep at nighttime. If you travel across time zones, your circadian rhythm will likewise be disrupted. Commit the green side to memory. It will help protect you when your circadian rhythm is thrown off.

***

✓ **Structured / Energized / Mineralized Water:** I explain what structured water is in detail in the Water Chapter. For now, it's enough to know that structured/energized/mineralized water more easily hydrates your body, whereas unstructured/demineralized water consumes a great portion of your body's energy to structure it so the cells can use it. When water is structured and mineralized, it has a negative charge and is in its natural state, such as water in nature (waterfalls, natural springs, rivers, etc.). Some fascinating studies suggest that structured water has antioxidant properties. See "Effect of Antioxidant Water on the Bioactivities of Cells," International Journal of Cell Biology, Aug 2017.

✗ **Destructured / Deenergized / Mineral-depleted water:** This is, in my opinion, the biggest factor for the poor health that is rampant around the globe. Water is so crucial it has its own circle in our model. As we will discuss in later chapters, water and minerals act synergistically to keep you healthy. When you remove one from the other, disastrous consequences ensue. Destructured, de-energized, de-mineralized IS depleted water.

***

✓ **Proper diet / Whole food:.** Your body only needs water, minerals, and salt on a consistent, continual basis. This might explain cravings and emotional eating. Hmmm? This very simple concept has been convoluted and confuses the public. Eat natural food! Real food! Eat anything that was on this Earth in our distant past. Water is key to so much of our health, and the water content of what we eat is especially important. Approximately thirty percent of your water comes from your food. Whole foods, whether meat, vegetables, or fruit, are what you want to consume. Processed foods do not contain water. Avoid them so that you aren't dehydrating yourself. Remember the first sentence, students? I'm biased toward a low-carb and carnivore diet because I've personally experienced tremendous health improvements from them.

✘ **Poor Diet:** This is self-explanatory. Processed foods, grains, excess sugar, and seed oils contribute to chronic disease because they activate all the red circles on the health wheel.

***

✓ **Exercise / movement:** Our bodies are designed to move. Yet, exercise *does not necessarily* lead you to lose weight. If movement doesn't help you lose weight, what does it do? The great news is that building and maintaining muscle is key to your longevity for a myriad of reasons. It balances hormones, produces more mitochondria, stimulates brain function, reduces cellular stress . . . the list goes on. AND, the more muscle you have, the more structured water your body holds. The more structured water your body can hold, the longer your longevity. Oh, and if you weigh more after weight training for a while, it's because muscle weighs more than fat. Why? Because muscle holds more water.

✘ **Sedentary Lifestyle:** When you don't use your body as nature intended, it causes inflammation in the lymphatic system (see the Movement Chapter). And a sedentary lifestyle has other negative effects. With less muscle mass from lack of exercise, your body isn't as efficient at metabolizing energy. Why? Partly because you have fewer mitochondria in your muscle cells.

***

✅ **Remove Toxins:** Go organic or chemical-free to decrease the toxic load on your liver. Our environment is full of toxins. It's in the air we breathe in the form of pollution and smoking. It's in the food we eat through fertilizers and pesticides. It's in the cleaning products in our home, the toothpaste we use, and the deodorant we apply. Even water is full of fluoride and other chemicals. Your body has to detoxify everything you put into it and expend energy and water to clear out toxins, and that hurts you in the long run. So spare yourself a lot of stress and live as toxin-free as possible.

❌ **Living in a Chemical Environment:** Proactively avoid manmade chemicals. If you have a lot of toxins in your environment (hairspray, nail polish, shampoo, or anything chemical), then your liver, as a detoxifying organ, has to metabolize all of these chemicals. Toxins cause stress on the liver, and more liver stress means less time you'll spend on the planet. Doesn't it make sense to reduce your chemical exposure?

***

✅ **Sun Exposure:** Adequate sun exposure is vital for your health. Vitamin D is synthesized in the skin by the sun. Sunlight and infrared light are critical for healthy blood flow. They increase structure to the already structured water in your cells, and the structured water is how cells communicate. The greater the charge separation and water structuring in blood vessels, the easier the blood flows, and *viola!* Lower blood pressure then occurs without the side effects. Remember, all the green lifestyle factors will help to lower blood pressure. **We all know this!**

✗ **Lack of Sun Exposure:** The truth is that sunlight is good for your health. What happens to your body when you live in a big city? Air pollution impedes absorption and limits your vitamin D levels…another reason to hate smog! Sunlight—and, more specifically, infrared light—helps the fluids in your body move. It reduces inflammation.

At this point, some of this might sound like gobbledygook, but everything overlaps and interconnects. Antioxidants donate electrons to other molecules that are missing an electron in order to make them stable. When molecules are missing electrons, they are unstable. Antioxidants thereby create stability all day, every day. The more structured water you have, the more of this benefit you have. The indirect effects of limited sun exposure, as when you are stuck in an office and don't absorb sufficient sunlight, can be quite harmful. All of this relates to the circles in the model. See why this model is so important?

✅ **Calorie Restriction / intermittent fasting:** The general public definitely misunderstands this factor. We are told that you have to eat every few hours to keep your metabolism "revved up." This advice is correct in a high-carbohydrate environment. Why? Because your fat-burning enzymes are dormant, and the only fuels readily available are carbohydrates or proteins. But logically, does it make sense to constantly work your digestive system to this degree? Why not give it a break and let it rest?

There are numerous reasons to restrict your food intake. Did you know that overeating and carrying excess weight can increase your risk of chronic disease, often compounded by snacking. When you avoid snacks, your insulin remains in check, and all the green circles hum along. Thus, your insulin won't spike and cause inflammation.

❌ **Excess Frequent Eating:** As mentioned above, every time you eat, you raise your insulin. Every time you put something in your mouth that isn't water, you have a response. Note that our bodies aren't designed to have insulin activated all of the time. Remember, our ancestors couldn't snack all day. They ate when they could find food. We are not meant to eat frequently, but if you are on a carb-based diet, that's exactly what your body tells you to do. You can't resist until you go through sugar withdrawals. No bueno.

***

✅ **Meditation / mindfulness:** Your mind, body, and spirit are all interconnected. You can control your mind, mindfulness, and physiology through meditation, which reduces stress. Your mental health is incredibly important. Why? Because thoughts and emotions control everything. Now that you are becoming a student of the model, you'll see that all of the pieces are beginning to fall into place. We have the answers to your health questions. Just stick to the green side.

❌ **Lack of Mindfulness:** Do these words describe you—unaware, conscienceless, mindless, clueless, ignorant, or oblivious? Well, after reading this book, you will be informed, educated, and equipped for better health. Question: What does that mean according to our model? Answer: A reduced chance of disease.

***

✅ **Grounding / connecting to nature:** Grounding is one of the most powerful antioxidants, period. Here is a video link that explains the power of grounding: youtube.com/watch?v=FxT5IqFP6P8. When you ground yourself by touching your bare skin to the ground, you expose yourself to the natural negative electrical charge of the Earth in the form of electrons. Electrons are the negatively charged particles of atoms that help to neutralize free radicals. What are free radicals? They are unstable atoms missing electrons. Add electrons, and you make them stable! Bingo! We just discussed this a couple of paragraphs before, and it bears repeating. Commit the model to memory!

✖ **Disconnecting from Nature:** When you wear shoes, you are disconnecting from the Earth. You are a biological robot and must ground in some way. Grounding recharges your battery. If you're not grounding, you're not getting fully recharged. There is an endless supply of electricity on the Earth. Connect to it! Think of it as "electrical nutrition" and feel free to explore a scientific study explaining the importance of this concept—"Integrative and lifestyle medicine strategies should include Earthing (grounding)," Science Direct, volume 16, issue 3 May-June 2020, pages 152-160.

***

✓ **Fulvic / humic acid supplementation:** One more reason everyone is overweight and ill is because the soil has been depleted. A few centuries ago, the soil was life-giving and fertile. Today, plants can't access the minerals in the soil because the microbes are being destroyed. Fulvic acid is extremely important because it is produced by microbes in the soil and gives nutrition to plants. It makes the minerals bioavailable in the soil, as in composting and cow manure. See the Food Chapter for a wider explanation of water, sunlight, fulvic/humic acid supplementation, and regenerative farming and how they all interconnect.

✘ **Lack of fulvic / humic acid:** Lack of fulvic and humic acids means you are not getting the minerals you need. All you have to do is take a gander at our model. One of the red side factors shows mineral deficiencies.

***

✔ **Reduce electromagnetic frequencies:** Avoiding EMFs is so important that I've already mentioned it in the opening chapter. Your body is an electrical system and runs on electricity: the membranes of your cells have voltage-gated channels (doors that open and close). The EMFs disturb these voltage-gated channels because they're unnatural frequencies. This has been theorized to lead to cellular stress. Do you see how it all fits together?

✘ **EMF exposure:** You might ask yourself, *Why is there exponential growth in gut disorders and autoimmune diseases?* Could it be because of massive amounts of electrical pollution, along with other negative lifestyle factors? I think so. After all, the quantity and intensity of exposure are the root of the problem. Some research suggests these frequencies are causing long-term harm.

Other Negative Lifestyle Factors to Avoid (Common Sense)

So many possible lifestyle factors exist that it would be impossible to discuss every single one. The Ultimate Health Model™ is designed to educate us about the most crucial topics. Here are a few more to consider.

✖ **Medications. Let me be clear:** The Pharma industry treats symptoms and is a godsend for those who will not follow the health model's green side. If you are stubbornly entrenched in the red side, then drugs can alleviate the pain and agony of fibromyalgia, gout, or whatever the disease may be. The truth is that some people aren't going to change. They will continue to manage their lives and symptoms through medications. And although medication might help to alleviate a particular condition, the side effects can be problematic. Why do you think they post warnings on medicine labels? (See the Molecular Nutrition and Food Research Journal's article, "Medication-induced mitochondrial damage and disease," on the NIH website—https://pubmed.ncbi.nlm.nih.gov/18626887/).

I believe that everything we need to heal ourselves

is provided in nature. In fact, medicines can make the red circles go around and contribute to disease. Manmade chemicals are not the answer IF you want to live on the green side.

✖ **Mineral deficiencies:** A lack of minerals links back to our destroyed soil. Cow manure puts minerals into the soil and helps produce healthy topsoil. This provides nutrients to plants and ends up in YOU. Look for mineral-rich sources and how soil is taken care of. Buy from knowledgeable, reputable farmers and co-ops.

✖ **Overuse of alcohol:** Too much alcohol is toxic, and the liver has to process the toxins. Why do you think alcoholics get fatty liver disease?

More About Healthy Hank & Heidi and Diseased Dan & Debbie

Before we delve into body design in the next chapter, I'd like to mention the characters presented in the model—Healthy Hank & Heidi and Diseased Dan & Debbie. I know this may seem odd, but these characters are going on the same journey as you are. You've seen Healthy Heidi & Hank and Diseased Debbie & Dan in the graphics; many readers can identify with them. In one way or another, each inspires us to improve our overall health either through positive or negative examples. I wanted to make this book a fun experience, not just another boring book telling you what to do with your health.

To find optimal health, you want to engage in lifestyle choices that create movement on the green side of the chart. If you struggle with chronic disease, it's because you engage in too many of the lifestyle factors on the red side. If you have questions about whether something in your life is contributing to optimal health or chronic disease, please get in touch. I'm always happy to help guide people through the Ultimate Health Model™ and determine whether a behavior lands you in the green or the red.

Now that you understand the basics of the health model, it's time to learn a little more about how the body functions and what that means for your health. We'll dive more deeply into other health factors in the chapters ahead. Right now, the important thing is to be aware that a better life awaits. If you follow the information in this book to its natural conclusion and test your lifestyle choices against the Ultimate Health Model™, you will feel better. You'll experience better sleep, lose weight, and improve overall health and vitality.

How could it not?

CHAPTER 3
Body Design

Just one living cell in the human body is more complex than New York City.
~ Linus Pauling

When I first started researching cells, what I learned blew me away. We are full of these miniature machines on a microscopic scale—trillions upon trillions of them. I started to wonder, *Is every cell in each of our bodies like a little person?*

Cells are complex and self-sustaining, each with a role to play. I compare stem cells to baby humans. I envision them growing up and maturing, just like we've gone through adolescence into adulthood. The sophistication increases. I suggest you respect your remarkable body and its cells and support it with your best efforts.

Communication Under Your Skin

The parts that make up the cell (organelles) can be thought of as parts of a factory or city, each with its own specialized tasks to perform. But they all have to communicate in order to make your body run. All approximately thirty-seven trillion of them.

I couldn't help but think that only eight billion people live on the entire planet. We can barely communicate with our neighbors, let alone the whole world. How in the hell are thirty-seven trillion cells communicating with each other? It's hard to wrap our minds around a number this vast. I want to graphically represent thirty-seven trillion because it is such a mind-blowingly big number: 37,000,000,000,000!

It's remarkable what our bodies are capable of and what we don't give them credit for.

I thought of my sister's cancer and my mother's. I thought about what we're designed to eat and how we're designed to live. As I researched more about the intricacies of the body's design, I no longer believed that cancer is a disease. It might, however, be a failure to communicate between the cells.

I theorized that cells that are by themselves mutate because they can't communicate with the rest of the body. My ideas do have merit. Recent research shows that the extracellular matrix (a combination of collagens, connective tissue, and proteins) is altered and dysfunctional in cancer cells. This matrix is how cells communicate with one another through electrical impulses, chemical messengers, and structured water. The membrane of the cells has hundreds of "satellite-type receptors" in the form of proteins, fats, and carbohydrates. This is called the glycocalyx, and it's fascinating to me. Interestingly, most doctors have no idea what this is.

Learning about the body's design showed me just how remarkable we truly are. We don't need drugs. We don't need to alter our chemistry. The body is a perfect biological machine on its own, and nature has endowed us with everything we need.

Over the years, I've changed a lot about how I interact with my body. I actually communicate with it regularly, and when I slip up, I tell it I'm sorry. I know it's listening to me. It's all connected, a gift that I have been given by God or the universe. Respect that gift, and you'll reclaim your health and live a long life.

The Power of Cells

The human body is more complex than most of us can imagine, and I am in awe of it. Understanding the design of your body allows you to work in harmony with it, creating a healthy biological ecosystem that protects you from illness and disease. When you see the puzzle pieces that make up our bodies and cells and the machines (in the form of proteins, fat, and carbohydrates) they create, you understand the perfection of the body's design.

The body is composed of only three macronutrients:

- Proteins: mainly the structural components; enzymes (molecules that allow biochemical reactions in cells) and hormones.
- Fats: structural components found in the membranes of all cells and organelles; an energy source in cells; a necessary vehicle for absorbing certain vitamins; a precursor to hormones and enzymes, and more. Vitamins A, E, D, and K are fat soluble. If you are on a low-fat diet, what do you think will happen? Why would you stress your body by denying it fats?
- Carbohydrates: an energy source and components of cells.

With this basic knowledge, you can start on your path to health and vitality.

When you don't understand the design of the body and cells, you risk putting stress on it, which can eventually lead to chronic disease. Ignorance isn't your fault, but it is within your ability to change.

Body design encompasses everything from your skeleton to your organs to your nervous system, but it all starts with the cell. Were cells designed by God? Did some alien species bring them to Earth? Maybe evolution happened and shifted us into the version of humans we know today. We may never know, but it's clear to me that the cell had to be created first because it's so complicated and intricate.

Here is some evidence I believe leans toward some creative force designing the cell. Take a guess at how many molecules are in a typical cell. One hundred? One thousand? Try one approximately 1 trillion! 1,000,000,000,000! Holy smokes! Now, guess how long it would take to count that high? One month? One year? Try 38,000 years! Double holy smokes! You would have had to start counting when the planet was gripped in an ice age and wooly mammoths were roaming the planet! These kinds of facts just boggle the mind!

We only know a small percentage of what cells can do. Cells are incredible powerhouses that operate your brain, your nervous system, your gut, everything. Individual cells grow and turn into tissues, then organs, and finally into different bodily systems such as cardiovascular or digestive. Each cell on its own is a self-sufficient, self-functioning unit. Each cell has a digestive, skeletal, respiratory, circulatory, and nervous system. That's remarkable to me. Cells are incredible: you only need one of them to form an entire organism, like protozoans and bacteria.

When I first started studying the human body, I

thought of cells as these tiny, simple things. In my mind, cells were building blocks that did nothing individually but were useful once aggregated together. As I did more research, I learned the truth: cells are the basis of all life. Your cells are constantly dying, regenerating, and replicating. Approximately three million cells in your body are generated *every second*. That equates to three hundred billion a day. Just sit and ponder that. Some last only a day, while others, like red blood cells, can survive for three months before they are replaced.

With that much variety and that much power, it's hard to imagine those cells were not intelligently designed.

The illustration in this chapter is designed to help you understand these organelles as analogous to a city.

The Design of Human Cells

Not everyone sees the simple power of cells. People say, "There's no design at work here. It's all evolution." I don't believe that's the case. I believe they were engineered. How could something so powerful just randomly form, out of the blue, morphing into the shape of a cell?

Let's look a little closer at exactly how cells work and what they do for the body.

The cell might not literally be a factory or a city,

but the similarities are mind-blowing. Every organelle in the cell has a unique purpose—a function it serves within the cell. Each of those organelles has several important parts that allows it to meet that function. Following is a list of some of the major organelles inside the cells and their functions:

- cell membrane
- mitochondria
- ATP synthase pump
- endoplasmic reticulum
- lysosomes
- peroxisomes
- cytoskeleton
- Golgi apparatus
- nucleus

Cell membrane: A lot of people think the nucleus is the brain of the cell, but it's the membrane that does the heavy lifting. It communicates with other cells by water and electrical charges. That communication is instantaneous. It's not "Okay, John's going to talk to Angela, and Angela's going to talk to Jesse" in a daisy chain. Billions of reactions are happening every second. As discussed earlier, the membrane is composed of the components that cells use to talk to one another. This complex array of proteins and lipids, both attached to carbohydrates, is cumulatively referred to as the "glycocalyx." Think of it as both a communicative device and a barrier or shield or a wall around a city. It keeps outside stuff out and inside stuff in. Emerging science in recent years now implies that damage to this layer is a causative factor in all diseases. Interestingly, keeping it intact is following the green lifestyle factors. See frontiersin.org/articles/10.3389/fcell.2020.00253/full as a resource.

Mitochondria: Think of the analogy of mitochondria as power lines in a city. The cell's mitochondria are the electric power plant that provides energy for the cell to do whatever its function is. When you metabolize food, whether carbohydrates or fats or proteins, it creates carbon dioxide, water, and adenosine triphosphate, or ATP (the energy currency the cell uses). The ATP is then transferred to different parts of the cell, fueling its needs. Also, think of mitochondria as thousands of batteries in the cells powered by water, oxygen, nutrients, and sunlight. Yes, in this analogy, mitochondria function as both power lines and batteries. Both move electricity. A famous scientist once said that life is " the orderly flow of electrons." Electricity is the orderly flow of electrons, and the microscopic batteries create this flow and, consequently, electricity. That's why mitochondria are one of the main circles in the model. Interrupted flow from dysfunctional mitochondria contributes to disease.

The mitochondria also help in the synthesis of hormones. They literally control whether a cell lives or dies. Cancer is an uncontrolled proliferation of cells. So, if the mitochondria are malfunctioning, you can see the possible connection to cancer and all other diseases.

A very interesting study was done by cancer researchers who took different cell cultures and injected mutated DNA from cell nuclei and mutated mitochondria. Yeah, mitochondria have their own DNA, and that's why they have their own circle on the model (because we love them)! The mutated mitochondria produced mutated cells, whereas the mutated cell nuclei did not.

ATP synthase pump: Although this pump is not an organelle in the cell, I mention it here because of its striking similarity to a man-made machine. Inside the mitochondria, the ATP synthase pump is the final step in producing energy from the electron transport chain (a series of very complex reactions that move electrons down a series of molecular machines). This pump is designed exactly like a machine: it has a flywheel, rotors, and even bearings.

Seeing that pump, I thought, *There's just no way this is not intelligent design. It's an impossibility. Evolution might impact how our design adapts over time, but how could this biological design look like a machine without any intelligence behind its creation at all?*

Endoplasmic reticulum: Each cell also needs to produce proteins, fats, enzymes, steroids, and whatever else the cell needs to run and stay alive. That is done through the endoplasmic reticulum. There's a rough endoplasmic reticulum and a smooth one. Together they form an assembly line, pumping out protein and fat-based molecules from the directions they receive from the cell's DNA. The DNA blueprint ensures they're creating the right proteins for the kind of cellular component they become. And this will become very clear in the cell graphic!

Lysosomes: When this assembly line makes a mistake, the cell needs to be able to wipe the slate and start again. The lysosome is the cell's recycling center. This organelle is acidic to break down this cellular debris. For example, if a protein is made incorrectly, such as being misfolded, or if the cell contains damaged proteins, the lysosomes break it down into its individual amino acids and send it back to the endoplasmic reticulum so that it can be made again.

Interestingly, these organelles also function as a sort of housecleaning service. When you fast short-term, the cells clean house and send these damaged, worn-out proteins and other damaged cellular components to the recycling bin. In essence, your cells clean themselves in a process called "autophagy" or self-eating. When you're constantly eating, the cells get full of garbage with no time to clean. No wonder this contributes to disease.

Peroxisomes: When you produce energy within the cells, that process creates free radicals, the pollution of the cells. These charged-oxygen molecules bounce around the cell doing damage, stealing electrons. The security and detoxification system in the cell is called the peroxisomes. Peroxisomes help to combat free radicals. One of these peroxisome enzymes—cytochrome p450—is altered and damaged by the active ingredient in herbicides and pesticides called glyphosate. Glyphosate is ubiquitous in our environment, meaning everywhere at once. An interesting fact about glyphosate is that it's designed to kill the microbiome in the soil, which is made up of bacteria, fungi, and protozoa. The mitochondria in your cells are actually an ancient form of bacteria that took up residence in living things in a symbiotic relationship. If glyphosate is designed to kill bacteria, then you understand the conclusion I'm drawing. We will discuss the importance of soil in later chapters. When you're in balance, the pollution in your cells is constantly being cleaned by the peroxisomes. When those systems are out of balance, you get an overabundance of free radicals, which causes inflammation, stress, dehydration, and all the other red side cellular circles in our model.

Cytoskeleton: You know that your body has a skeleton. Well, so do your cells. The cytoskeleton is made of protein fibers called filaments. The cell has hooks called integrins that work like scaffolding to hold the protein fibers together. It looks remarkably like it was built by humans, just like we would build a house or a cathedral.

Golgi apparatus: This is where the newly formed "biomolecules" (cell components) are sorted, modified, and processed before either being used by the cell or exported out of the cell to other parts of the body. It's the Post Office in the graphic. Look at it as a sorting system. Isn't that remarkable?

Nucleus: This is where the DNA is stored in chromosomes. The DNA is the "blueprint," or code, of how to make the various parts of the cell. The language and syntax of DNA is frighteningly similar to the computer coding we use today. When you start to reflect on these concepts, it's hard to imagine there wasn't some design involved in this.

Cell charge: The final piece of the puzzle is the cell charge. Once again, this isn't an organelle of the cell, but it is vitally important in cell design so that cells maintain a negative charge at all times, between -30 and -70 millivolts. When cells are replicating, the charge could be as high as -150 millivolts. When the charge starts to move into the positive, that's when chronic disease can start to develop.

Electrons help your cells maintain their negative charge, and the red side lifestyle factors contribute to decreasing the negative charge of the cells because it's causing inflammation. As we talked about earlier, electrons aid in the antioxidant process. Did you know you don't need to consume exogenous (manufactured outside the body) antioxidants? Your body makes them in the form of glutathione, uric acid (pee!), and melatonin, to name a few. We'll discuss melatonin in more depth in the Sleep Chapter. Like discussed earlier, an orderly flow of electrons is what you want. The green side encourages this, and the red side discourages it.

All of these parts of your cell work together, a stunning cooperation without which our bodies wouldn't work at all. I can't help but think of the mind-boggling similarities between cells and the computers we all use today. Are we biological robots? Cells are where it all starts—but they aren't where it ends. Your body has all kinds of safeguards in place to protect these marvels of engineering.

One important way the body protects itself is through your immune system. This remarkable system is what keeps you protected from viruses, pathogens, and infections. White blood cells are one of the main players in this incredible orchestrated process. They are the body's defenders or superheroes. As we learned from our model, when this system is suppressed from the negative lifestyle factors, we are more prone to chronic disease. Sugar is public enemy number one for the immune system.

Sugar in high concentrations is damaging to the body, so cells lock the door and don't let sugar in. Instead, they redirect sugar to your red blood cells or to your endothelial cells (cells that make up the innermost layer of blood vessels). Some studies and research estimate the average American consumes a half pound of sugar a day. That's a whopping one hundred fifty pounds a year! How incredible that 200 years ago, we were consuming approximately four pounds a year.

Redirecting sugar works in small doses, but if your sugar levels get too high, your red blood cells start to become inflamed or glycated (sugar-damaged). That's what a hemoglobin A1c test measures: the glycation of the red blood cells. The sugar also damages the endothelial cells, the cells in your blood vessels. Having an "aha" moment? Excess sugar isn't your friend.

Evolutionary Design

I believe we are designed to consume animal products, with few plant products. This is an anatomical and anthropological perspective. Anatomically, we have very low stomach acidity, in the range of pH 1.5 to 2. In contrast, a cow's stomach is approximately 5. Why would we need such an acidic environment for digesting plants? Moreover, cows have four compartments in their stomachs (often referred to as four stomachs). Why? It's so they can digest plant material efficiently into bioavailable nutrients. They chew the cud, regurgitate, and eat continuously all day long. Maybe cows and other ruminant animals were put here for that reason: to be able to take undigestible plants and turn them into food for humans.

Doesn't it make sense that they are a conversion machine for us? We have one stomach, not four. That's how ruminant animals make themselves incredibly nutritious for us. The microbes in ruminants ferment plant materials in an incredibly complex way. When humans eat plant material, we ferment it too. But we don't have four chambers in our stomachs. We aren't designed to eat a lot of plant materials. Here's an eye-opener. Cows chew for eighteen hours a day. Do *you* want to chew your feed for eighteen hours a day? I have things to do!

The amount of nutrition in plants is not enough. Most of our plants have been hybridized today. There was no such thing as broccoli back in the day. Potatoes had more fiber and less starch back then and plants were more fibrous, too. Apples were not as big, not as sweet. And our ancient ancestors ate meat because they didn't get enough nutrition from plants. You must add fiber if you don't eat meat. The same goes if you are consuming only a Westernized diet of ultra-processed foods. This is simple biochemistry. After all, the microbes in your gut need something to eat, and they will feast on three things—fiber, ketone byproducts, or YOU (your mucosal gut lining). BUT with carnivore and protein-based diets, the microbes won't feed on you. Instead, they will feed on the metabolites from ketone production. Now do you understand why you might be having leaky gut problems?

Also, our colon (where a majority of plant fermentation happens) is very small. Same question: Why would it be so limited if it weren't because we should consume limited plant material? Anthropologically speaking, researchers have determined through bone testing that our ancestors ate mostly meat. They discovered this using nitrogen-15 testing. This measures a specific nitrogen isotope in the bones to determine how much protein is being consumed.

Your Hemoglobin A1c

Do you know your hemoglobin A1c score? This test gives you a score out of 100. Below 5.7 is normal. Between 5.7 and 6.4 is considered prediabetic, and 6.5 or higher in two separate tests is considered diabetic. In layman's terms, you want a low score.

Glycation is the process of sugar molecules sticking to something else in the bloodstream or something in the cells. It's a process that shares electrons and becomes a very hard bond to break. It's obviously damaging to the body.

The "Maillard reaction" describes this. Heat basically alters the sugar molecules, and that's what you see with the browning effects of sugar. That's a form of glycation. A piece of toast is an example. Remember that toast is sugar in the form of carbohydrates. Interesting side note: A1c only measures glucose glycation, not fructose. That's a big deal when approximately 80 percent of processed food contains fructose. Once again, my Ultimate Health Model™ describes this.

With this information in hand, it's obvious that sugar, *not* saturated fat or cholesterol, is one of the main contributors to chronic disease. The other dietary factors are seed oils (which I personally believe are the absolute main player) and refined grains. We will discuss these "evil three" in more detail in later chapters. Chronic disease? We just need to think about it logically. Why would cholesterol cause inflammation and metabolic problems when sugar is the substance coating your red blood cells?

The Randle Cycle

Sometimes, fat in excess can be bad for you—when you eat it *in combination* with sugar. What do we do as a society eat at every friggin' meal? We mix carbs and fats together! Think about your last breakfast. What was it? Eggs and bacon with orange juice and toast? When you do that, the sugar and the fats compete for oxidative phosphorylation, which means they're both trying to be metabolized in the cells at the same time. This process is known as the Randle cycle (or the glucose fatty-acid cycle), named after a scientist who discovered this phenomenon in the early sixties. I find it shocking and disturbing that some medical professionals don't know about this crucial process in the cells. This ignorance manifests in hospital menus and hospital cafeteria services. Giving hospital patients pudding? WTF?

This process happens in the cells constantly, to different degrees, and that's why eating either a vegan or a carnivore diet puts less strain on the cycle in which your cells are preferentially burning either carbohydrates or fats. When people say, "Saturated fats cause heart disease," they are looking at it in a very reductionist way. It is way more complex and complicated than that. Suffice it to say, like our model states, if it causes chronic cellular oxidative stress or unhealthy cells, you can be sure it's contributing to disease.

Isn't it interesting that carbs and fats aren't found together in sufficient amounts in nature, except for milk? There is no other.

That's why when you go on a vegan or low-carb diet, you often lose weight and start to regain your health—not because the fat or meat was bad for you (or the vegetables and fruits), but because you're not activating the Randle cycle.

We'll talk more about what food is actually good for you and how to balance your diet in Chapter 7. But it's hard to completely divorce the subjects of food and the design of your body. Just think about how much your gut health impacts your overall health and vitality. That's because of your microbiome.

Your Microbiome

A microbiome is a collection of bacteria, fungi, viruses, protozoa, and other microbes. You have microbiomes across your body, including your lungs, your skin, and your gut. Scientists know more about the surface of Mars than they do about our microbiomes. But what we do know is fascinating.

Take, for instance, your skin's biome. Your skin itself is divided into three layers:

1. An acid mantle
2. A lipid bilayer, often described as the natural "oil" in your skin
3. The skin tissue also called the epidermis

The microbiome lives inside the acid mantle and acts as a barrier to prevent infection from entering the body. When you wash your skin using harsh chemicals and soaps, you destroy the lipid bilayer as well as damage the delicate acid mantle. That dries out your skin and can lead to infection and inflammation.

That's what eczema, psoriasis, and other skin diseases are—they're most likely rooted in our favorite word, inflammation. It's your body responding to you washing your skin or hair and damaging your microbiome, which is designed to protect you from pathogens and foreign invaders. Your skin is your first line of defense, so it makes sense not to damage it. Remember, though, from our model, that eczema could also be exacerbated by any of the red lifestyle factors. It's this circular relationship that is key to understanding the model.

What about the biome in your gut? Did you know that you can't technically digest fiber? The microbiome in your gut does it for you. It's incredibly important to have a healthy, balanced gut microbiome, but too often, our diets and lifestyles put it out of whack. Again, this is where the connection between food and your body's design becomes impossible to tease apart.

Interestingly, it's not necessarily about having a diverse microbiome. It's about having a balanced one. Studies show that strains of bacteria can have multiple functions. If one particular species is absent, another can take over its duties. That might explain why some people thrive on a meat-based diet while others do well on a plant-based diet. In contrast, the diet that will put you "six feet under" quicker than you might like is the SAD diet (standard American/Western diet). This diet is loaded with the big three or what I like to call the triad of demise—sugar, seed oils, refined grains/flours. Isn't it interesting these three things, along with water, can make anything from a doughnut to a pizza crust?

When you eat sugar, seed oils, and refined grains in excess, it causes an imbalance in the microbiome in your gut. The metabolites created from digesting these "poisons" cause many issues—not only gastrointestinal but systemic throughout your body. After all, everything is connected. Millions of strains of bacteria exist in your gut, and they're creatures of habit. You literally train them to feed on these "toxins," and I use that term purposely. It's like your microbiome starts to say, "We're eating these poisons whether you like it or not, and you can't resist it."

When you change your diet and lifestyle, you change the microbiome, and those pathogenic cravings fade as the related bacteria die off. You're left with a microbiome favorable for digesting a proper human diet: one that consists of animal products, fruits, and vegetables.

The detoxification process can be challenging—

think of it like withdrawal from a drug. At first, those pathogenic bacteria will be desperate, starving for the nutrients they've been trained to expect. But after a month or two, they start to die off, and the cravings vanish. Your microbiome starts to heal, returning to a state of equilibrium and balance. It starts working for you instead of against you. Chronic inflammation goes down all over your body, and those feelings of fatigue and general sluggishness will start to disappear.

We are talking only about the gut here. If these microbial communities are everywhere in the body, think of the ramifications of making them happy. The green-side lifestyle factors will help in this respect.

The body's design is truly remarkable, and it's up to us to take care of ourselves so that our bodies can work at peak optimization. One way to take care of your body is through grounding.

Grounding a Negative Charge

Grounding is connecting to nature. It's the process of bare skin touching the earth. Just like sun exposure, this increases blood flow. Why do you think walking barefoot on the beach or grass feels good?

The earth is a limitless repository of electrons. So when you ground yourself to the Earth, you get these electrons. Also, in nature, plants emit molecules that are beneficial to humans. The Earth is an electrical system too. How mind boggling to view the body as a huge electrical system connected to the dirt beneath our feet. We need to maintain a negative charge at all times. In fact, it's sort of like us… but on a huge battery.

Unlike humans, the Earth emits a frequency called the Schumann resonance, which is around 7.83 hertz (meaning 7.83 cycles of a wave per second). The harmonics of that frequency retune and recalibrate your cells to promote cell health, cell regeneration, and cell well-being. It also emits negatively charged electrons. What did we talk about earlier? Everything is based on the orderly flow of electrons. Now you can see the connections.

We said this earlier, but it's worth repeating—when you ground yourself, you absorb those negatively charged electrons through your skin. Those charges are like electrical nutrition the body needs in addition to food.

Your Body's Charged Systems

A negative charge also helps your blood flow freely and smoothly. How? The red blood cells have a net negative charge, thereby repelling each other. How is this accomplished? All healthy cells, including red blood cells, have a net negative charge. This is because all cell membranes have the glycocalyx layer, like we discussed earlier, as well as a negatively charged structured water layer in the membranes.

Think of the water layer as an adhesive material and a Teflon coating that glues the "phospholipids" (parts that make up the membrane) together. The more positive the charge in your blood vessels, the higher the possibility of red blood cells clumping together and making your blood thicker. You know what else happens when you thicken the blood? Blood clots! Chronic dehydration and all the red circles on our model contribute to this condition. What's a free way to get this improved blood flow? Once again, our model comes to the rescue! Engage in factors on the green side and restrict factors on the red side. It's that simple!

Why do you think doctors prescribe blood thinners? The thicker your blood, the harder it is to pump through the body. This causes cellular oxidative stress. It's amazing to me how you could throw a dart at a dartboard of chronic disease and hit something. Some very interesting views by Dr. Paul Mason made this clear to me in a presentation he gave on LDL (low-density lipoproteins, one of the carriers of cholesterol), which will be discussed in later chapters.

Basically, he said heart disease is most likely contributed to by oxidized or damaged LDL. How does it get damaged? From all our negative lifestyle factors. This, in turn, contributes to blood clots and our "I" word — inflammation.

Getting back to grounding, the best part is that it's completely free and accessible to us all. The Earth itself has an endless supply of negatively charged electrons in the microbiomes of its soil and groundwater. It's the greatest antioxidant of them all. All you have to do to access it is to touch the ground.

I don't have the benefit of living in an area where nature is easy to get to. But luckily, you don't need to go to the forest or the ocean to practice grounding. I sit in the park where I live, ideally with my bare feet in the grass or on the dirt. I try to spend twenty or thirty minutes grounding every day, but of course, life happens. The longer you're grounded to the Earth, the better, but anything is better than nothing. Waterfalls and beaches are also a great source of these electrons. You can dip your bare feet in the water and ground that way. Understand that just being in nature is exposing you to these incredible health benefits.

Anecdotes and studies abound of people who cure their back pain or even arthritis when they start regularly grounding, all because their body's charge was so off.

Here are more ways for you to ground:
- Anytime you're on the Earth, whether that's sand, soil, or even rock and gravel, take your

shoes off and walk barefoot. Your shoes have rubber soles that insulate you from the Earth, so make sure to take them off. You can also sit and touch the ground with the palms of your hands.

- Gardening is another great way to ground yourself. Consider joining a community garden if you don't have a house with a yard.

- You can buy grounding mats to sleep on (see the recommendations page on my website, ultimatehealthmodel.com/recommendations). Negative charges travel through a wire to you. It's not as good as touching the Earth directly, but you receive a slow trickle charge all night long, which is great. Hey, just like charging an electric car, right?

Grounding reduces stress and inflammation, boosts your immune system, increases hydration, and brings you good health. Funny—aren't those the cellular factors on the positive model? Yes, and you can start practicing grounding today. You can even head outside right now and give it a try. When you ground, you take control of your health and reclaim your power.

Another great way to relax and reduce stress is through your breathing. When was the last time you stopped and thought about how you breathe?

Now that you've learned about the cell and its

many complex functions, see the following illustrations that compare the cell to a city with a key for explanation.

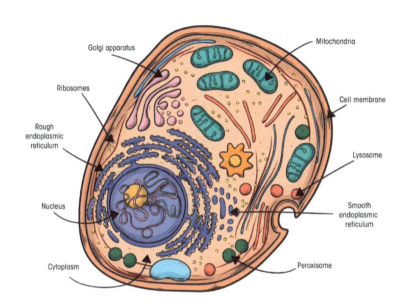

WHY ARE YOU SICK?

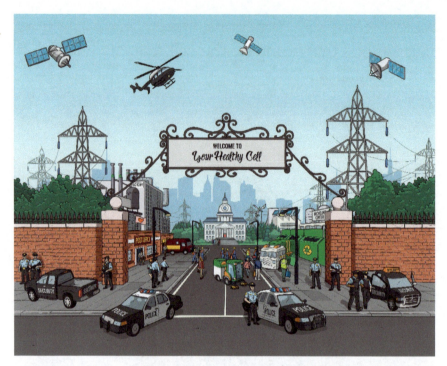

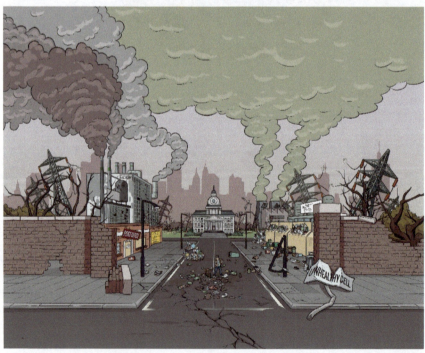

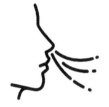

CHAPTER 4
Breathing

Only those who know how to breathe will survive.
~ Pundit Acharya

At the top of Chapter 2, I mentioned that the most important lifestyle areas and factors are **breath, sleep, water, food, movement, environment, and thoughts and emotions**. Let's start by taking a deeper dive into breathing.

You've probably heard the saying, "You only have a limited number of heartbeats before you expire." Well, the same goes for breaths. Use them wisely! You'll understand this concept as we work through this chapter.

No More Mouth Breathing

"Dude, your nose is whistling."

That was the constant refrain of my childhood. I was always stuffed up. Every time I tried to breathe through my nose, there it would go: *tweet t-tweet tweet*. Tired of being teased, I started breathing through my mouth instead. I spent years thinking, *As long as I'm breathing, it doesn't matter how I breathe. Right?*

Fast forward two decades, and I discovered the work of George Catlin and the journalist James Nestor. Catlin theorized that mouth breathing causes inflammation, which leads to dehydration and a host of other health problems. *Have I been doing this wrong my entire life?* I wondered.

I was determined: no more mouth breathing.

If only it were that easy to make the change. My sinuses were so stuffed that breathing through my nose felt like an impossibility. But I was angry. I was determined. I was tired of that voice in the back of my head saying, "Dude, your nose is whistling." I wasn't going to listen to my fear. I was going to shut my mouth—at any cost.

When I first started, I could barely force air through my nose. Determined and dizzy, I stuck at it as much as I could, ignoring that painful whistle. At first, I breathed shallowly, getting just enough air to make do. But I knew that the stakes could very well be life or death. I stuck at it, and slowly I could breathe a little more. And a little more.

Week by week, my sinuses cleared. My nasal passages opened, and that mocking whistle vanished—for good.

After just two months of nose breathing, I found that my allergies had completely vanished. My nose was so clear that when I got COVID-19, I didn't even get stuffed up, let alone lose my sense of smell, which was a common symptom. I slept better. I was healthier. I didn't wake up with a dry mouth or headaches.

I was furious that doctors hadn't told me how important nose breathing was. How could they not know something this important and critical to the body's homeostasis? I had changed the shape of my jaw and narrowed my airway, breathing through my mouth all those years. I wasted decades never being able to breathe right, afraid of that whistle. I also suffered needlessly from headaches, gut problems, and asthma.

But I'm grateful, too. I'm grateful that the body is so resilient. Even after fifty years of damage, it was able to heal itself when I learned a better way.

The Dangers of Mouth Breathing

Why are you sick? One factor is habitual mouth breathing. Don't worry, though. It isn't too late for you to change how you breathe.

Nose breathing is a must! Chronic mouth breathing is detrimental to your health because it leads to a lessening of oxygen being released from your red blood cells and to the tissues. This leads to many problems, including chronic inflammation. In contrast, nose breathing solves this problem, along with others, because it brings in more oxygen to the tissues, not less.

When you learn to breathe through your nose, you completely change the way that your body uses oxygen. You become less dehydrated and reduce your overall inflammation. Your nose is a filter without imperfections, and using it will help you reclaim your health and vitality. This amazing organ serves more than thirty functions. It purifies, sterilizes, warms, humidifies, and pressurizes the air before entering the lungs. It prepares the air. Mouth breathing offers none of these benefits.

Let's look at the damage mouth breathing can do, the benefits of breathing through your nose, and how to change your habits to get healthy.

People think, *I'll breathe through my mouth so I can get more oxygen in. The more oxygen I breathe, the better off I'm going to be.* That's completely wrong. Interestingly, the reason you breathe at all is to release carbon dioxide. But when you mouth breath, you exhale carbon dioxide too rapidly. Your body has more than sufficient amounts of oxygen dissolved into your blood circulation: up to ninety-nine percent in some healthy individuals and as low as approximately ninety percent in individuals with breathing disorders. That's only ten percent, but makes a vast difference.

Here's what really happens when you breathe through your mouth.

Your red blood cells are the transport system for oxygen and carbon dioxide throughout the vasculature. Every time you breathe in, you take in oxygen. Every time you breathe out, you release carbon dioxide. The problem is that when you breathe through your mouth, you end up overbreathing. Most people breathe (in and out) about twenty times per minute instead of the ideal six or seven times.

When you over-breathe, you're allowing too much off-gassing of carbon dioxide. In other words, when you mouth breath, you exhale carbon dioxide too rapidly. The red blood cells need that buildup of carbon dioxide to help release oxygen from the hemoglobin in red blood cells. They compete for space. Why do you think people are told to breathe into a paper bag when they're hyperventilating? To increase carbon dioxide levels!

This depletes your blood of carbon dioxide. Contrary to popular belief, carbon dioxide is not a useless waste product. It is actually vital to the oxygenation of the body's tissues. The body needs carbon dioxide to release oxygen from red blood cells, oxygen that is needed by the body's tissues for metabolic functions.

In addition to slowing down breathing, nose breathing properly prepares the air you inhale by acting as a filter while humidifying, pressurizing, and warming the air you breathe in. Mouth breathing has none of these benefits and actually irritates and inflames our lungs with cold, dry air, causing the lungs to create mucus for hydration.

When you breathe less (from the diaphragm) you allow the oxygen to penetrate the deeper lobes of the lungs for more efficient oxygen exchange. That's also why people tell you to calm down and take a few deep breaths when you're stressed or anxious. You can't be relaxed and anxious at the same time.

Mouth breathing creates a low-oxygen environment called hypoxia. Hypoxic conditions are absolutely toxic to your body. Hypoxia contributes to type 2 diabetes, gut issues, Alzheimer's, heart disease, rheumatoid arthritis, osteoarthritis, and, of course, cancer. A cell can turn cancerous within forty-eight hours of not receiving oxygen. That's it.

Why? Because hypoxia causes cellular oxidative stress and all the other negative circles in our model. This is all one big puzzle, and when all the pieces fit together, you'll see the bigger picture. That's how important oxygen is to your body.

Mouth breathing also contributes greatly to dehydration, and we'll learn more about the importance of hydration in Chapter 6. For now, it's enough to know that dehydration leads to stress, inflammation, and all other red circles shown in the Ultimate Health Model™. When you breathe through your mouth, you lose forty percent more moisture than when you breathe through your nose. That dehydration also contributes to wrinkles through glycation of the collagen proteins in the matrix of the epidermis. You might be saying to yourself, *Damn! My mouth breathing is contributing to that crepey skin on my arms?* Yep.

Plus, when you eat a lot of carbs, especially refined carbs, it causes inflammation that can plug up your nose. When you can't breathe through your nose, you end up breathing through your mouth instead—and that contributes to weight gain. Why? Because of inflammation. Everything is related. That's another reason breathing through your nose contributes to weight loss. Keeping your mouth shut is the secret the weight-loss industry doesn't want you privy to. Can't make money on the advice to keep your mouth shut!

You were never meant to breathe through your mouth. That's why you have a nose.

Your Nose Knows the Way

Your nose is one of the most important organs in your body. It is the most complex filter that exists—humans have never come close to creating something so intricate. It bears repeating that your nose filters the air, warms it, and humidifies it all at once. It sterilizes the air and sends it to the lungs properly prepared. Think of your lungs as delicate organs that can be easily damaged by inflammation and the nose as the guard protecting them. Breathing through your nose is critical for your health! I can't emphasize this enough! Here are just some of the benefits:

- **More oxygen:** When you breathe through your nose, the nasal system releases nitric oxide. This gas dilates your blood vessels, opening them up and allowing them to take in more oxygen. More oxygen, happier cells.

- **Deeper breathing:** When you breathe through your nose, you breathe from your diaphragm, which gets the oxygen deeper into your lungs. The bottom of your lungs has more of the alveoli (the oxygen/carbon dioxide transferring sacs) that carry the oxygen into your blood. Think of these alveoli as little balloons. If you damage them, they won't inflate properly.

- **Weight loss:** Fat primarily leaves the body through the breath. That's because fat is partially composed of carbon dioxide. A small portion might be excreted through the kidneys and excrement, but the majority is breath. Did you know that some doctors and dietitians, as well as fitness trainers, don't know this? That is pretty alarming, considering some people put their health decisions in these professionals' hands. When you eat carbohydrates (made up of carbon, hydrogen, and oxygen), your body turns them into carbon dioxide, water, and ATP energy. Then you breathe out the carbon dioxide. You're releasing the fat and moisture in the form of water! When you breathe through your nose, you literally lose weight.

- **Nasal cycle:** Your nose naturally cycles air between nostrils. One takes in more air than the other; they alternate approximately every thirty minutes to four hours. When I learned of this, I was literally floored! The amazement once again of the human body! This process helps to regulate your parasympathetic nervous system (rest and digest) and sympathetic nervous system (fight or flight). If you breathe through your mouth, you don't benefit from this incredible adaptive and homeostatic process.

- **Filtering, sterilizing, humidifying properties:** Let's get a little gross and talk about boogers. Some people flick them, others eat them (gross), and some think they are a nuisance. Boogers actually protect your health. Your nose hairs have a sticky mucus lining that traps pollutants in the air. And that's what boogers are. Dried mucus with pollutants. So next time you pick your nose, thank your boogers for protecting you. Something else to consider . . . I implore you to nose breathe, especially if you live near freeways, rail yards, or industrial areas. Numerous studies show that people who live in these areas have a higher risk of all chronic diseases for the reasons mentioned.

Now, I'm going to go off into the weeds and show you just how connected and interrelated all bodily processes are. Most of us have heard of SIBO (small intestinal bacterial overgrowth). Millions of Americans suffer from this condition. Some symptoms mirror IBS (Irritable Bowel Syndrome). These include abdominal discomfort, bloating, constipation, and diarrhea. What if I told you this was related to chronic mouth breathing? If you're bloated and feel gassy, maybe you should consider changing your diet AND your breathing habits. Your body is telling you something is wrong.

Yep. Basically, in a nutshell, this is what happens: Water and carbon dioxide are the first steps in creating the stomach's hydrochloric acid and gastric juices. We know from this chapter how mouth breathing affects water and carbon dioxide levels in the blood. Low stomach acidity doesn't allow full breakdown of food particles, and they can start to ferment in the stomach and proliferate bacteria. This is passed onto the small intestine, where bacteria counts are low because this is where most of the absorption of nutrients (carbs, fats, proteins) occurs. Higher bacterial counts will start to feed the bacterial biomass and not the host (you!) Bacteria will die in the small intestine and create endotoxins—and WHAMMO! INFLAMMATION!

I give this long explanation so you understand this connectivity and how you can relate it to ALL other health ailments.

You may be wondering, *What about exercise? I can't breathe through my nose while I'm exerting myself.*

You can, actually. It takes some doing, but you shouldn't be exercising any harder than you can while still breathing through your nose. Start small. If you can do only ten jumping jacks while breathing through your nose, that's great. Start there. Tomorrow you might find you'll be able to do twelve, and then even more.

There are some caveats here. Understanding the difference between chronic and acute stress is super important. Chronic stress leads to chronic inflammation, while acute stress and inflammation lead to adaptation and, in turn, make the body more resilient. So mouth breathing on occasion is beneficial.

The bottom line is that unless you're eating or talking, keep your mouth closed!

Control Nighttime Breathing

We should be breathing through our noses, not our mouths, even when we sleep! When I first switched to nose breathing, my health hugely improved. Encouraged, I decided to go further. I knew I could tape my mouth shut at night to stop mouth breathing, but I was scared. What if I choke? What if I die?

But breathing through my mouth was literally killing me. I grabbed a piece of tape and taped my mouth closed. I figured that if anything happened and I panicked, it would be easy to get off.

In the morning, I felt incredible. My mouth wasn't dry. I felt better rested. It was immediately obvious that mouth breathing had been ruining my sleep.

One night, about a year after I started taping, the tape came off in the night, and I started mouth-breathing. I immediately woke up with a pounding headache. My throat was dry and scratchy, and my nose hurt. I put a piece of tape back on, and within a few minutes, the headache was gone.

You might be wondering about the snoring epidemic out there. Why? It's because your mouth is open at night. Wiping that drool off your pillow in the morning is a sure sign. Believe me, I was also there.

To find and purchase mouth-breathing strips, please visit the recommendations page on my website at ultimatehealthmodel.com/recommendations/. To learn about how to safely tape your mouth shut, see the strategies at the end of this chapter.

Think of nose breathing as a balancing act for your body. It keeps everything in sync and impacts all of your organ systems. In fact, the negative impacts of mouth breathing go even further than we've discussed so far. Are you ready to see just how much damage your mouth breathing is doing?

A Damaged System

The profound effects of mouth breathing are wider than you might realize. It isn't your fault that no one has explained them to you. But once you know, you'll be on your way to better health and vitality.

Allergies / Asthma: When you breathe through your nose, the air is prepared for your lungs in all the ways we discussed. It is filtered, hydrated, and warmed. Keeping your mouth shut protects the delicate tissues of your lungs. When you breathe through your mouth, you get none of those benefits. The air goes in your mouth along with pollutants and contaminants. The body creates mucus to trap those particles. Also, mucus is created as the body tries to moisturize the tissues.

Again, what does this cause? Our favorite word: inflammation! The damaging effects of dehydration cause the blood vessels in the lungs to constrict in order to hold onto moisture. An interesting study on the deleterious effects of pollution on your health demonstrated that particulate matter in the air had potentially damaging effects on your high-density lipoprotein (HDL) and low-density lipoprotein (LDL). These are the buses that carry the cholesterol around the body, causing them to oxidize. Asthma is also rooted in mouth breathing—no question. Want to get rid of those money-sucking and, frankly, chronic disease-contributing other-the-counter or prescribed allergy pills? Keep your mouth shut!

Chapped lips: It's no surprise that breathing in and out across your lips is what causes them to chap. You're dehydrating your lips with every breath. Throw away that balm and start breathing through your nose.

Sleep apnea: When you have sleep apnea, your tongue relaxes and falls into the back of your throat. Every time that happens, you lose oxygen through a narrowing or complete blockage of your airway, and it can happen as much as fifty times a night. The resulting hypoxia makes the body think it's dying, so it releases stress hormones like adrenaline and cortisol. This, in turn, activates all the negative cellular factors in our model. By the way, guess where the first place in your body gains weight? The tongue.

It seems like everyone is being diagnosed with sleep apnea these days. They sell you a machine that forces air into your lungs for thousands of dollars instead of just helping you breathe through your nose. When your mouth is closed, your tongue doesn't fall back because you naturally rest it on the roof of your mouth and don't choke. As simple as that.

Nightmares: Did you know that mouth breathing might bring on nightmares? When you mouth-breathe, you lose oxygen, and your body thinks it's dying. Could this be translated as a signal into your brain of bad dreams? I believe so.

Tooth decay and gum disease: Mouth breathing contributes to everything from tooth decay and gingivitis to gum disease. Saliva controls the acidity in the mouth, maintaining the pH level in a normal range. This helps to balance the microbiome in the mouth. (Yes, every organ and tissue in the body contains microbiomes.) Think of it like mouthwash. When you dry out your mouth by breathing through it, you disrupt this delicate balance, allowing pathogenic bacteria to multiply.

Facial deformities: Mouth breathing as a child can contribute to crooked teeth, long face syndrome, and sunken chins. This adverse effect of breathing incorrectly really pisses me off. Sucking my thumb misaligned my teeth. This is a phenomenon that is rarely discussed and discounted to genetics. This is doing a great disservice to all the young children whose development is still biologically active. *Please* let them know the importance of this.

George Catlin first documented the phenomenon in the 1800s. He was a lawyer who quit his job to become a photographer and focused on the local indigenous people. As he took hundreds of photographs, he noticed differences in the faces of North American indigenous people and his own British colonists. He noticed the Native Americans had strong jawlines and perfect teeth while the Europeans were not so lucky. Most people assumed the differences were genetic. Wrong! Catlin noted that the Native Americans he was photographing always kept their mouths shut.

Fascinated, Catlin saw that his subjects rarely showed big facial expressions, and they covered their mouths when they were laughing. They kept their mouths shut at all times, other than when they were eating or drinking. White people, on the other hand, often breathed through their mouths. Catlin became one of the first myologists—scientists who study faces. Even two hundred years ago, Catlin knew the importance of correct breathing: "The air is not suitable for the lungs without first being filtered," he is documented to have said.

Chronic inflammation: One of the big contributors to inflammation is mouth breathing. We can see the proof through studies showing that people who have sleep apnea have a higher risk of chronic disease. Why? Because of all the red cellular circles we discussed in our model—all of them being players in this disharmonious symphony.

With all these ill effects, it's a no-brainer that we should all be breathing through our noses. Doing so just requires a little bit of effort and attention.

Breathing for Relaxed States

Dr. Sarah Hornsby, a myofunctional therapist, shared with me the importance of nose breathing. In our conversation, she told me, "The most critical aspect of switching from mouth to nose breathing is the ability to get the body into a more relaxed state."

"When we nose breathe," she said, "we activate our parasympathetic nervous system or our 'rest and digest' response. When we mouth breathe, we automatically activate our body's 'fight or flight,' or sympathetic, stress response."

Dr. Hornsby continued, "The importance of this concept begins to make more sense to people when they think about sleeping and breathing through the mouth. How are you supposed to sleep well if your body is stuck in a fight/flight stress response state due to poor breathing?"

Strategies for Nose Breathing

Keep your mouth closed. It really is as simple as that.

But if you're wondering what else you can do, don't worry. Strategies exist to help you move toward better health through nose breathing.

In India, a yoga uses the fire breathing technique to stimulate nose breathing. To do that, you just have to sit or stand comfortably. Push on one nostril to seal it, and breathe in and out five times. Then switch sides. Close the other nostril and breathe in and out five times.

This kind of breathing helps you regulate and balance your systems and gets your body used to breathing through your nose. It's especially helpful if you're really stuffed up and have a hard time nasal breathing on your own.

Another important strategy is taping your mouth shut at night. I've told you about my own nose-breathing journey. Don't be an idiot and tape your mouth shut with duct tape. Instead, use skin-safe mouth strips. Then you don't have to worry about suffocating. You aren't taping your mouth *closed*. Skin-safe mouth strips have a small hole in the middle to allow breathing in emergency situations. As stated in earlier chapters, we will make recommendations for products we endorse. The mouth strips I suggest are from SomniFix.

Make sure that you get in some practice nose breathing during the day *before* you try taping your mouth shut. If you struggle to breathe through your nose at all, it's advised you clear the congestion by getting your nose back in sync during the day like I did, and then you can move on to nighttime routines.

If you don't like the idea of taping your mouth, look into a chin strap that holds your jaw in place at night but lets you open your mouth if you need to. The important thing is to remember that you're sleeping for about eight hours a night—that's a huge portion of time. Even if you nose breathe all day, you're losing so much progress every night if you fall back into mouth breathing.

Sleep is a huge part of our health, and getting a handle on it is incredibly important. That's why sleep is the subject of the next chapter.

WHY ARE YOU SICK?

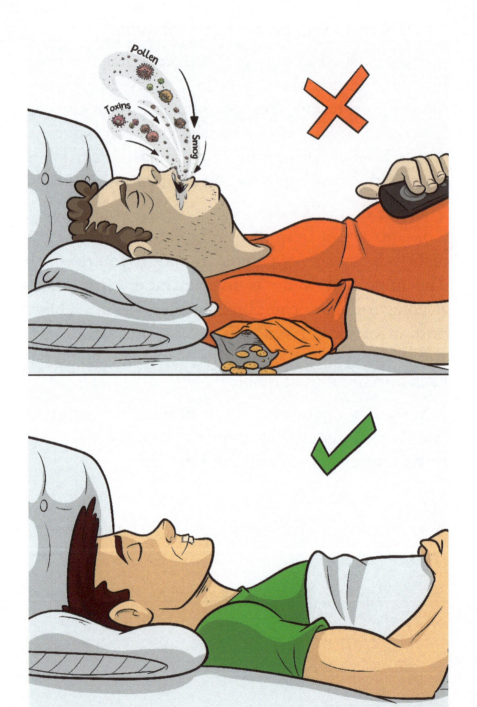

What has to be taught first, is the breath.
~Confucius

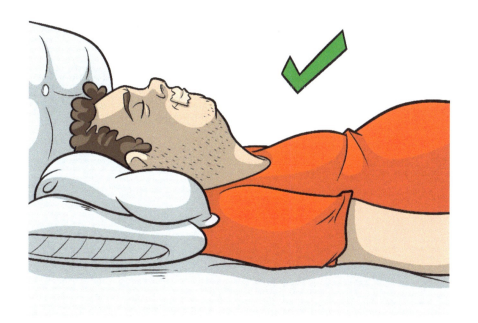

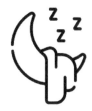

CHAPTER 5
Sleeping

Without enough sleep, we all become tall two-year-olds.

~ JoJo Jensen

Sleep is vital to regulating ALL functions in the body.

For example, our body is designed to follow circadian rhythms, patterns of behavior, and function based on the time of day. Examples are metabolizing food or repairing and restoring cells and tissues. When we have non-restorative sleep or not enough sleep, some of these crucial functions are disrupted.

Additionally, for those who regularly work at night, some of these metabolic processes are driven by darkness, such as producing melatonin. Melatonin is a major antioxidant in the body which helps fight free radicals and regulate hundreds of the body's functions. I theorize that melatonin is also produced from all the green lifestyle factors. It's the *circadian rhythm disruption* that is detrimental to health and contributes to chronic disease. This is why people who work night shifts may be prone to chronic disease and being overweight. The point is that the melatonin is certainly important, but I believe it can be derived from various sources, whereas the circadian rhythm cannot be produced by other factors. You can't change day to night. That's an immutable fact. If you're up at night, you're up at night.

Without sleep, you can't do anything—your body literally shuts down. I've seen that firsthand.

In 2008, I drove to LA to visit my parents. I was stressed out the night before, going over last-minute trip details, and I only got three or four hours of sleep. Over the course of the eight-hour drive, my brain started to fog over. The endless freeway stretched on and on, and I felt my eyelids grow heavy. I turned the music up loud, trying to stay awake.

I finally reached my exit and breathed a sigh of relief. I had made it.

I turned the wheel, intending to make a gentle exit from the highway, but my fogged-over brain couldn't navigate the off-ramp. My perception was off, and my tires hit the median before a rush of adrenaline jolted me awake. Narrowly avoiding a deathly crash, I righted the car and took the exit.

My palms were slick with sweat, and my heart was beating so fast I could feel the reverberation in my chest. *Oh my God*, I thought. *That was almost it.*

My parents didn't live far from the exit, and I decided I was safe enough to finish the drive. All that adrenaline had definitely woken me up. But just in case, I slapped my face, getting my blood flowing, and rolled all the windows down so the cold air would keep me alert.

I was lucky to survive that day. Without sleep, your body literally stops functioning. I liken it to the analogy of "your body's software short circuits." You're not doing a "virus scan" just like a computer, and so it shuts down. Eventually, it will force you to sleep—whether you're in your bed or driving a car. If you want to reclaim your health, you need to understand the importance of sleep. When you do that, you understand how beautiful the system of your body is and what a miracle of design sleep is.

Sleep Governs Everything

We, as Americans and most of the world, are chronically sleep-deprived. It's a damn epidemic! Everybody was freaked out about COVID, but no one talks about this silent killer that indirectly kills more people than you can possibly imagine. Not to scare you but to make you aware!

Sleep is a huge factor in your overall health—more important than diet and exercise *combined*. Getting good sleep every night can add decades to your life. Bad sleep? Well, it can subtract the same amount. And you *thought* sleep was something you could forgo if cramming for a test or a late night at work!

Sleep is your body's opportunity to heal and repair. Imagine your body operating on itself: when you're asleep. It's like you're under anesthesia, and you're the surgeon doing the important work to reset your systems, clear cellular debris, and replace damaged and diseased cells. Your body literally paralyzes your muscles—a process called muscle atonia—so you don't move around. Have you ever experienced sleep paralysis? That's a misfiring where your body wakes up, but your brain is still sending the signals to your muscles to relax.

Your body uses sleep as an opportunity for your cells to heal, rebuild, and repair. If you don't sleep at night (yes, it has to be at night, more on that later), your immune system is suppressed by as much as thirty percent. This is also when your muscles heal and rebuild. If you work out every day and don't get enough sleep, it will be significantly harder to build muscle mass. You're doing all the damage but not giving your body time to heal and grow.

Note that sleep and grounding together recharge

your body. You sleep to reset and update the body's software. Grounding recharges the battery. The electrons come through your body. That's wireless electricity restoring your battery. That's why you should ground every day and look into purchasing grounding products. See the Recommendation page on my website.

A lot of people push their bodies past the point of safety like I did when I nearly fell asleep at the wheel. But at the end of the day, sleep always wins. You either fall asleep at the wheel, or you pull over and take a nap on the side of the road. You have no control over whether or not you fall asleep.

What you *do* control is the quality of the sleep you get. All sleep isn't created equal. You need to learn how to make your sleep as restful and healing as possible.

Because if you don't? The consequences are a killer.

Life or Death Consequences

When I was in my twenties, I stayed up all weekend partying. And I do mean all weekend. Once, I went a full forty-eight hours without sleep.

It's fine, I told myself. *I'll sleep when I'm forty. It doesn't really matter.* I had no idea how much damage I was doing to my body. Sure, I had a hangover from lack of sleep. I felt sick. But I just pushed the feelings away. I let it pass.

Now, I'm more in tune with my body. If I don't sleep, I feel horrible. My ears start ringing. I feel like I'm drunk. My eyes glaze over, and I have trouble concentrating. My digestion isn't optimal, and my body aches. All because I understand the damage I'm doing, and I'm tuned in enough to recognize the signs. In a society that runs twenty-four hours a day—and more importantly, a culture obsessed with and addicted to their electronic devices—it's no wonder people sleep only four or five hours a night, every night. And whether they know it or not, they suffer the consequences of that decision.

Knowing more about how sleep works is the first step toward understanding its importance and starting to change your own sleep habits. Let's look at five big myths around sleep and the truth behind them.

Myth #1: The brain and the nervous system are needed for sleep.

The brain controls all bodily processes, so it's understandable to assume, "Oh, that's needed for sleep."

Understandable but wrong.

All living things sleep, regardless of whether they have a brain or even a central nervous system. Why? Because all cells exhibit a resting state. Take plants.

Plants have a type of internal clock, or "circadian rhythm," that tells them whether it's night or day. Like many people, plants are less active at night. It might not be asleep in the traditional way, but it's a form of rest that allows them to heal and rebuild. Maybe the secret to healthier plants is to hum "Rock-a-Bye Baby" to them.

Even hydras, single-celled organisms that live in the ocean, sleep. Researchers from Kyushu University in Japan and Ulsan National Institute of Science and Technology in South Korea tested hydras and found that they took on different shapes at different points in the day. In certain shapes, their metabolic activity went down—they were engaged in a form of sleep.

Scientists believe sleep is an evolutionary process that started long before brains had even evolved. Since sleep is how restoration and repair happen, it makes sense that every living thing has to be able to enter that state.

Myth #2: Sleep is only related to brain waves and brain function.

Now that we know the brain isn't necessary for sleep, it's probably obvious that sleep and brain function aren't as intimately related as some studies suggest. Organisms that have brains allow for more complex functioning, as stated earlier, but a brain isn't required for sleep.

To reiterate this very important concept, every cell has evolved with a mechanism called circadian rhythms. This is the body's biological clock. It keeps you awake in the daytime and asleep at nighttime. Thanks to their circadian rhythm, cells are programmed to do certain things at night and other things during the day. They might metabolize food and build proteins during the day, and recharge or rebuild or repair cell components at night. If you do the wrong activity at the wrong time, it throws your cells completely out of balance by disrupting these rhythms.

For instance, your cells are designed to metabolize nutrients during the daytime. If you eat meals at night, even if you do it regularly, it causes chronic inflammation. Wow! Our favorite word again. By now in the book, you are starting to see these inseparable relationships between these circles on the model.

This is one of the challenges of night-shift work. Even if you think your body has adapted to a different schedule, your cells are still programmed by millions of years of evolution with their specific circadian rhythms. That's why so many night-shift workers experience poor health. The good news for people who have to work into those wee hours is that our friend, the mighty mitochondria, also produce melatonin (sleep hormone), which isn't circadian rhythm dependent. Also if you have to work these grueling hours, please incorporate as many of the green lifestyle factors as possible to mitigate that pesky chronic inflammation.

Myth #3: You can change your circadian rhythm.

Our ancestors rose and slept with the sun. Thanks to modern technology, we're no longer stuck on the sun's schedule. But that might not actually be a good thing.

Our bodies have a set circadian rhythm, and there's absolutely nothing you can do to change yours.

Almost no one sleeps all through the evening and night—even I don't do that. There wouldn't be enough hours left in the day. Besides, most of us need only seven to nine hours of sleep, and the sun can be down for a lot longer than that. But the fact is that our bodies are designed to sleep for a good portion of that dark time—and not to sleep during the day.

We think our bodies can adapt to new schedules given enough time, but the truth is that while we might adapt mentally, our cells never do. We make melatonin starting approximately around 10 p.m., peaking at 2 a.m. and lasting until 4 a.m. If you're awake for all or most of that period, your body isn't producing sufficient melatonin.

You may know that melatonin helps you sleep, but it's also an antioxidant. As mentioned earlier, it's one of the major antioxidants you produce endogenously (within your body). While it is produced at night, it's also produced in the mitochondria, independent of night or day. In addition, it's derived from ultraviolet light and exercise. I theorize this is the reason night shift workers are not dead. I believe everything on the green side helps make melatonin and mitigates the chance of getting chronic disease.

So give the mighty melatonin the credit it deserves! It is crucial to regulate metabolic functions in the cells.

Myth #4: Sleep is a waste of time.

I went to Reno in the fall of 2022 to hang out with a good friend. On that Saturday night, I slept only four hours. The next morning, I had a pounding headache. But more interestingly, I was ravenously hungry. And I never feel hungry.

Sleep deprivation influences and disrupts your metabolism through two hormones: leptin and ghrelin. Leptin is your satiety hormone, while ghrelin is your hunger hormone. Lack of sleep disrupts the balance of these hormones and makes you feel hungry even though you might be full. What's causing the hormone disruption? Possibly chronic dehydration. Just look at the model and it will help you out.

That's just one part of why every single person should be sleeping for seven to nine hours a night. Studies show that losing just a single hour of sleep a night causes problems ranging from overeating to loss of concentration. Chronically sleep-deprived individuals are in a zombie state most of the time, and their quality of life suffers as a result. Did you know that top athletes and entertainers prioritize sleep? It helps them perform at the top of their game.

If you're sleeping only five or six hours a night, you really need to take into consideration how important sleep is to your overall health and well-being. Would you rather spend that extra hour getting that report done, or catching up on the latest TV trend? Or would you rather contribute to your health and gain an extra, say, *twenty years* to do anything you dream of?

Have you ever heard someone say, "I'll sleep when I'm dead." Well, you'll be dead a lot sooner if you get inadequate sleep.

Myth #5: Nothing stops cancer.

Most of us think the only way to stop cancer is to blast it with radiation, cut it out, or poison it. The truth is a lot more surprising: cancer cells can be interrupted with melatonin.

Like discussed earlier, every cell in your body has a circadian rhythm, and cancer cells are no exception.

Melatonin inhibits the enzymes that cancer cells use to reproduce. Without that enzyme, cancer cells can't get nutrition and can't reproduce. They're basically on pause while your body is producing melatonin.

When you're awake during the time when your body is programmed to sleep, cancer cells might be doing their terrible work twenty-four hours a day, not just in the waking hours. That means cancer progresses and spreads faster, and it's another reason why sleep is so important. Please, if you know someone currently battling this condition, educate them on this connection. I so wished I had known about this when my family members were diagnosed.

Myth #6: Only the brain produces melatonin.

Nope, wrong. Again, I shot a buzzer. *Beep!* Liver and muscle cells also produce melatonin, and most other cells as well.

Conventional wisdom says the pineal gland in the hypothalamus is the master regulator of melatonin, according to Veronique Greenwood in a 2021 article in *Quanta Magazine* entitled "Sleep Evolved Before Brains. Hydras Are Living Proof." Interestingly, though, this gland produces only a fraction of the melatonin, approximately five percent. The bulk of melatonin is produced intracellularly. That's why if you read melatonin levels in blood, it isn't an accurate measurement. Guess what manufactures melatonin in the cells? The mitochondria. If you have "dysfunctional mitochondria," what are the unfortunate results? Isn't this model amazing? You just throw a dart and *boom!* You hit something.

With those six myths tackled and debunked, you're ready to learn how to change your poor sleep habits. The great news is that healthy sleep is possible for all of us. The first step is to learn what stops healthy sleep and start to avoid those things. The second step is to make positive changes to embrace healthy sleeping habits.

Let's start with the habits you want to avoid.

Healthy-Sleep Stoppers

All kinds of things might be stopping you from getting a good night's sleep. Those include stimulants, sleeping pills, inflammation, and sleep apnea, among others. *Aha* moment! If you put chronic insomnia into the disease banner on the red side, you have got your answer. This model is almost spooky as to what it can predict.

Stimulants: We all know the dangers of stimulants like caffeine and energy drinks. When you drink a stimulant-containing beverage to help you stay awake, it floods your system with adrenaline. Why do you think your heart starts racing? It makes you jittery and gives you false energy to keep you awake. But in the long term, that's stressful on the body. It causes inflammation and chronic cellular oxidative stress. And what does this contribute to? You can write this ending by now!

Sleeping pills: On the other side of the spectrum, you have sleeping pills. Everybody is popping these like they are candy. The problem is that sleeping pills don't actually help you sleep. They're sedative-hypnotics, which means what they're actually doing is sedating you—and sedation is not the same as sleep. You're unconscious, but you're not going into a deep state of restorative, reparative sleep. You're still getting some, but not enough. Most of us have heard of REM (rapid eye movement) sleep. That is not achieved with drugs. That's why people on sleeping pills often wake up groggy, still feeling as if they haven't slept. This one is hopefully a wake-up call (no pun intended), not to mention that medication is on our red lifestyle factors. Please understand that medications are a lifesaver for people who choose to live on the red side. Another lightbulb moment!

Chronic inflammation: Inflammation causes all kinds of sleep problems. Once again, we are using inflammation as a generic term. Please understand, and I can't emphasize this enough, that all the cellular and lifestyle factors on our model impact sleep. If you're eating too much sugar, if you're stressed out, if you're not drinking enough water, if you have type 2 diabetes, cancer, or heart disease—all of that causes inflammation. The older you get, the more influence these factors tend to have, which is why older people often don't sleep as much.

Diet's Impact on Sleep

By now, if you're understanding the model, you can start answering your own questions.

People who don't sleep tend to gain weight. That's because you're interrupting your metabolic processes. Excess sugar in your diet also disrupts sleep. Why do you think most kids aren't metabolically unhealthy? Because they don't have decades of built-up inflammation, which means they generally sleep better than adults. If you're not sleeping right, you're likely to gain weight, period.

Sleep apnea: As we discussed in the breathing chapter, sleep apnea stops you from dropping into true regenerative, reparative sleep. How does this happen? As you lie there, snoring away, the body is constantly going into a state of oxygen deprivation multiple times a night because your airway is getting obstructed. This triggers the body to release cortisol as well as a complex series of reactions to deal with the crisis. This causes inflammation. And like a broken record, we know what that causes.

Chronic dehydration: Even though all the red lifestyle factors contribute to chronic insomnia, I think chronic dehydration is one that's overlooked. Chronic dehydration depletes your tryptophan stores. Tryptophan is an essential amino acid you need to obtain from your diet. Tryptophan is one of the precursors to melatonin production. See where I'm going with this?

Ways to Improve Sleep

Luckily, you can improve your sleep in these surefire ways:

First, consider the hours when you're sleeping. Evolutionarily, when the sun goes down, you go to sleep. That's obviously not practical for most of us, but don't worry. The important thing is to be sleeping when your body is producing the majority of melatonin.

I go to sleep at ten at night and get up around seven each morning. You could sleep from 9 p.m. to 6 a.m. or from 11 p.m. to 8 a.m. The most important thing to remember is that melatonin production occurs, as I mentioned, between midnight and 4 a.m. If you go to bed at 1 a.m., that's a whole hour without melatonin production. A good rule of thumb is not to go to bed any later than 11 p.m.

With the "when" settled, it's time to think about the "how." Your sleep environment has a huge impact on your quality of sleep. Total darkness is optimal, especially from artificial light. Streetlights, clocks, TVs, and phones all interfere with melatonin production, even through your closed eyelids. Noise can also impact your sleep quality. Some people like to fall asleep to the sound of a TV or a white noise machine, but consider a timed shut-off so the noise doesn't continue all night. It puts stress on your body and could possibly stop it from entering a relaxed sleep state. Once again, try to implement as many green lifestyle factors as possible. This will definitely improve your sleep quality and quantity. You can hopefully say goodbye to those artificial hypnotics that might be causing harm, as our model shows.

If you wake up in the middle of the night, try not to open your eyes. Any artificial light will trigger your melatonin production to stop. Instead, try to stay still and see if you can fall back to sleep. Moonlight and starlight won't interfere the same way, but unless you're camping, you'll probably seeing artificial light somewhere in your bedroom.

If you're still struggling to sleep after doing those things, try to make going to bed into a kind of ritual. This turns it into a habit and helps make it feel like a natural part of your day. Take a hot bath or a shower right before bed. Go to sleep at a certain time. Whatever works for you. An important part of this is de-stressing. Try to calm your mind and stop its constant chatter. I know this is difficult, but try relaxing before entering dreamland. It will help greatly.

Sometimes, this advice can feel intimidating. Sleep

is so delicate that you don't want to do anything to disrupt your current habits. But remember that if you're not sleeping well or deeply for at least seven hours, those habits might actually be hurting you.

In our modern society, it's so hard to unplug. I'm not immune—I sometimes use my phone right before bed. I get it. Don't feel like you have to completely transform your sleep habits overnight. Start with baby steps. Invest in blackout curtains so there's no light in your room. Set a two-hour timer on your TV so it isn't blaring all night. Every step you make toward better sleep is a step toward better health.

Some habits are easier to take on than others. In the next chapter, I talk about water and how drinking structured water is one habit you *definitely* want to get into.

WHY ARE YOU SICK?

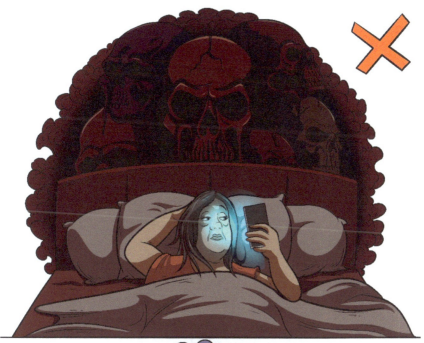

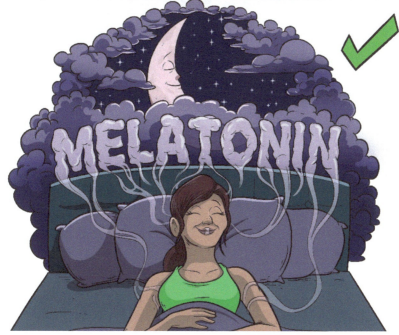

My mother told me to follow my dreams, so I took a nap.
~unknown

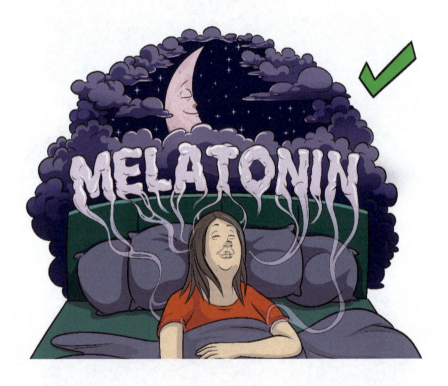

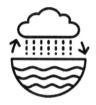

CHAPTER 6
Structured Water

Water is the lifeblood of our bodies, our economy, our nation, and our well-being.
~ Stephen Johnson

All biological information is probably stored in water. Everything from the beginning of time is most likely stored in water. Water is everything. As far as I'm concerned, water is all there is with a couple of other elements thrown in for good measure.

You can find a hundred books on how to lose belly fat in thirty days or what to eat to feel great. But none of them talk about our factors. Not one has mentioned the importance of energized structured water and its impact on our health. Ask twenty people, and only one will likely know what the term "structured water" means. Let's define it since you are probably scratching your head and wondering.

Understand that there is no formal definition of what structured water is. However, I'm using the term as it helps us understand how water "works."

Structured water is water found in nature. It's the water in lakes, rivers, and the oceans. This type of water gets mineralized as it passes over rocks and percolates through soils. Structured water is water molecules bonding and forming geometric shapes and structures. The shape determines the function. Everything on the green side of our model will help structure water, and everything on the red side will potentially destructure it.

Here's an example. Water is a liquid crystal, and diamonds are solid crystals. Diamonds are made of carbon. Your pencil lead, graphite, is made of carbon. Why does one bring in millions of dollars and you can buy the other for 25¢? It's because of the structuring of the carbon atoms. The pencil lead is not structured. But the diamond has a very complicated, intricate structuring (a lattice-like pattern).

Likewise, water is also structuring, with molecules coming together and breaking apart at approximately a billion times a second, creating information in the body. Imagine that! That's the software in your biological robotic body, and it's mindblowing.

Oh, by the way, think of your windshield in the

rain or going through a car wash. The water meanders down the window like a stream, zigzagging left and right without any right angles whatsoever. It never flows at right angles. Same for your blood vessels and the fluid streaming through them, like rivers in your body. These are forms of structuring and relate to everything in this chapter. Bear with me, and I'll explain.

The spinning action (or vortexing) of the water flow creates a crystalline structure in the water. Anything in nature will help structure the water. As I mentioned, anything we are doing on the green side will help structure it as well.

An Epiphany on Water

It's easy to take water for granted. I used to. I drank water out of the tap, or from bottles, and it tasted fine. It's water, right? It's just sort of . . . there.

In 2014, I dated a woman who drank spring water, delivered in large bottles to her house every week. I was surprised by how much better it tasted than the water I was used to. Could there be more to water than I imagined?

Feeling curious, I started to research water. I watched a documentary called *The Miracle of Water*. What really stuck with me was the mystical nature of water. I remember one scientist remarking, "Water might be the world's most malleable computer."

When I started to investigate this theory, I realized scientists are currently researching ways of using water molecules as computing devices. Water is a liquid crystal, just like the crystals in modern computers. ("Xrays indicate that water can behave like a liquid crystal," Science Daily, August 11, 2020)

It all started to make sense. Since humans are mostly water, we all are basically giant computers. So is your dog, so is a tree, and isn't that interesting? I saw that water was the key to life. I began to explore the potential impact of structured water—the natural water that exists in the world all around us. Structured water? WTF? Most people have never heard of this, and skeptics claim it doesn't exist. In nature, water molecules "structure" around minerals. Why are we constantly told to stay hydrated and make sure we get our electrolytes? Because electrolytes are "charged minerals."

This is why consuming water without minerals (reverse osmosis, purified, distilled) is *no bueno* long term. The water will leach minerals out of bone and tissues to balance itself. Remember that water needs minerals to perform all bodily functions. I started to understand that structured water is possibly able to hold information. Soon, I was drinking mostly structured water.

Before we go into a deep dive on the magical and mystical properties of water, let's first discuss dehydration. Everyone knows what that term is, but not many people know that your phone, and this darn thing I'm typing on, is also contributing to water loss. All you have to do is look closely and reluctantly at the model. Damn model, you're ruining my favorite pastime!

Chronic unintentional dehydration is a contributing factor to *all diseases*, period. Your migraine headache is caused by inflammation. What is the main cause of inflammation? Dehydration. Gut issues like irritable bowel syndrome (IBS) and Crohn's disease? Dehydration. Burn this into your brain! A scientist you might want to research for more thorough explanations of chronic dehydration and its detrimental effects is Dr. Batmanghelidj. Reading his books on water will blow your mind!

Let's quickly discuss the myths around hydration:

Dry mouth: This is false. By the time you are experiencing this, the body has lost a significant amount of water. Understand that only a two percent drop in hydration can cause cognitive impairment.

Any fluids will do: This is also incorrect and has caused the public much unnecessary suffering. Juice, soft drinks, coffee, and tea do not substitute for pure water. Yes, they contain water, but the sugars and stimulants actually have the opposite effect, causing more inflammation and dehydration.

Water is water: Wrong! This is a myth spread by

marketers. Water needs minerals to conduct bodily functions. When you consume purified, reverse osmosis, or distilled water, in which the minerals have been stripped, the unfortunate consequence is the leaching of minerals from tissues and bones for the water to perform its functions. Think of bottled, purified, and filtered water just like shitty processed food! This water is also processed and devoid of life-giving and life-sustaining properties. You can eat the cleanest, healthiest diet you want, but if the water you're drinking is "dead," your actually contributing to disease. Just like the model says!

Everything in life revolves around water. All biological, chemical, and enzymatic reactions in the body happen in water. Fun fact: Did you know that these reactions are far more efficient in solutions of low viscosity like blood plasma? Guess what makes the blood plasma thicker? Dehydration and all the factors on the red side! Another WTF moment! I understand some people don't like the taste of water. What they don't like is the "flat" taste of the water. The flat taste is when water is stripped of all its minerals, such as reverse osmosis or purified. This is because the minerals give it the flavor. We will discuss options to make your water taste better at the end of the chapter.

What I want to get across is that you want to make water your best friend. I know this sounds corny, but this concept is going to greatly improve your health.

The last point I want to make, before we get into the weeds about the social behavior and the energetics of water, is this (as previously stated):

The body needs three nutrients on a constant, continual basis: **water, salt, and minerals.**

If you forget everything else, remember that. Heck, tattoo it on your arm if you have to. This explains emotional eating, why people have cravings and much more. Remember, we're talking about natural salts like sea, Himalayan, or Celtic varieties—not table salt, which is chemically processed, refined, heated, and destroyed. It's no wonder this toxin causes high blood pressure.

Convincing others of the power of water and its structuring capabilities is challenging. Some people call it "foo-foo water" because they are so caught up in the traditional modes of thinking and just can't break through.

You could say I'm obsessed with water. I'm going to pose an interesting question. Why is it that Earth is seventy percent water and so is the human body by weight? Coincidence? I think not. But this can be misleading because by volume, our bodies are ninety-five to ninety-nine percent water molecules. You have to differentiate between weight and volume to do a true comparison. The water molecules are small and don't weigh much.

The Earth has an intricate system of rivers and

streams. What's the correlation to the body? Blood vessels are like the rivers, and the capillaries are like the streams—another mind-blowing tidbit to ponder. Did you know a water molecule is approximately twenty thousand times smaller than a red blood cell and sixty thousand times smaller than an average cell? I thought you might want to nerd out for a second!

Then, in 2019, my mother passed. I began to think a lot more about water—and its impact on the cancer that had taken her from me.

Gregg Braden, who wrote *The God Code: The Secret of Our Past, the Promise of Our Future*, found that the signature of our Creator is within our DNA. The phrase "God internal within us" is written on our cells in a computer-type code. I began to wonder: Is DNA a biological computer program? As I thought about water in the context of Braden's research, I had a powerful revelation:

What if he means that we are all water, and God is water, and God is consciousness? By deduction, water is consciousness.

Everything clicked into place.

You can't kill water. Energy can only be transformed, never destroyed. This is a very simplistic view of the first law of thermodynamics of physics. My mom and sister weren't gone. They're water, somewhere in the cosmos. I was relieved, knowing that I hadn't truly lost them. They're part of this larger water system and consciousness around all of us.

But I was angry too. Hell, I was furious! Cancer has taken so much of my family, and I believe cancer is caused by a miscommunication between the structured crystalline water within us in a very complex process. Is it possible energy in the form of photons goes into the structure of the water, gets to a cancer cell, and is interrupted? What if the water within us that isn't structured is causing disharmony? Could it be causing disease, just like a computer short-circuiting? This latest research is fascinating, confirming what we are discussing. (Structured Water and Cancer: Orthomolecular Hydration Therapy), (Journal of Cancer Research Updates, 2023,12, 5-9).

If the doctors had given my mother and sister structured water, they might be alive right now. But they're not.

No one is really talking about structured water. Why? Maybe it's because water's energetic and social behavior is way more powerful and important than it being a medium to dissolve "stuff" in. Water, in fact, is very difficult to measure and quantify. Not to mention that water responds differently to everyone. This is why when a water sample is analyzed in a lab, the results can be quite different than its counterparts in nature because of hundreds of different factors.

Few people understand the truly magical powers of water. I'm going to change these outdated views, starting right here, right now. Why are you sick? Water is a big answer.

The Powerful Truth of Water

Modern culture doesn't respect water. Some people don't respect it because they don't understand it. And that's a shame because water impacts every facet of our lives. All you consist of is mostly water. When you understand that water is everything and appreciate water as a living thing, you'll be more aligned to reclaim your health. Without that understanding and the ignorance it brings, you are not able to use this vital, life-giving resource to its full potential.

When a child is born, his or her internal ratio can be as high as eighty percent water by volume. As an adult, inflammation and dehydration push that ratio down to near sixty percent—and in old age, it's as low as fifty-eighty percent by weight. Why do you think a baby has silky skin that bounces back like a rubber band and an older individual's skin looks like a parched desert landscape? A perfect analogy is a full water balloon. A baby is a full water balloon, and your beloved grandparents are deflated water balloons! This is according to a 2019 *Healthline* article titled "What Is the Average (and Ideal) Percentage of Water in Your Body?" written by James Roland and medically reviewed by J. Keith Fisher, MD. Those numbers seem powerful—don't they?

They're actually a distraction.

The truth is that approximately ninety-five out every hundred molecules in the human body are water molecules. Is it any surprise that water has such a profound impact on our health?

Water has been studied extensively. At its core, it is incredibly simple: two atoms of hydrogen and one of oxygen. What we rarely study is the energy of water. Water molecules connect because they have different charges: the oxygen atom is negatively charged, and the hydrogen atoms are positively charged. This type of molecule is called a polar molecule, and that's what allows it to connect to other water molecules, forming shapes and patterns. The hydrogen and oxygen molecules' arrangement in structured water is predominantly hexagonal (six-sided, crystalline structure), while it's predominantly pentagonal (five-sided) in destructured (still or urban) water. Remember, this is all theoretical and based on what we know.

Hexagons are one of the most important shapes in nature. They're everywhere: snowflakes, beehives, snake scales, even insect eyes. Hexagons are incredibly efficient because they leave no empty spaces when they fit together. A hexagon is perfect for infinity. When water is properly structured, it forms these perfect hexagons, and that allows it to be something truly remarkable. I believe it to be the information carrier of the universe. Understand, though, that these aren't static shapes and patterns the water molecules are forming. This process is happening billions or more times a second. Ponder that!

Water Holds Memory

Consider this quote by Lucy Larcom: "A drop of water, if it could write out its own history, would explain the universe to us."

That statement is mindblowing to me. One drop of water? Are you friggin' kidding me? And some people think there is no order to the universe!

Water is a liquid crystal that can receive (entrain), store, amplify, transmute, and transmit information. It's the same reason that computers contain crystals. When light energy in the form of photons flows into these water crystals, the fitted hexagonal shapes allow information to flow uninterrupted. When the water isn't structured, the photons of light flow in, but are most likely interrupted. Recent advances in optic and water science are proving this to be true. The more "light" you lose over your lifetime, the quicker your demise. What causes you to lose light? The red lifestyle factors! By now, hopefully, you are model "experts."

The structure of water gives it an incredible power: information storage. Every single drop of water contains 1.5 *sextillion* molecules, according to "Calculating the Number of Atoms and Molecules in a Drop of Water," an article by Dr. Anne Marie Helmenstine, a science writer at ThoughtCo.com. Thanks to water's hexagonal shape, the different patterns connect to one another almost infinitely. That means what water can store and create is nearly infinite, too. Researchers and scientists hypothesize that the arrangements of these patterns might make up a type of alphabet.

The Intelligence of Water

Robert Gourlay, who has been a water scientist for thirty years, tells us that water is the highest form of consciousness: water, then microbes, then plants, then animals. Humans come last because we rely on water, microbes, plants, and animals to live and to receive their consciousness.

A very interesting set of experiments have been conducted on water, showing that water may be consciousness. One such experiment was done by Japanese scientist Dr. Masaru Emoto. Basically, he froze water droplets and then either used positive or negative emotions when talking to the droplets. The results were fascinating. The ones that received positive emotions like love and gratitude were perfectly shaped, beautiful snowflake patterns, while the ones that received the negative messages were deformed and misshapen. Even pleasant or violent music had the same effect. Could this be the reason negative emotions contribute to disease?

When you think about water as an intelligence that stores its own history, you begin to question our relationship with water.

For instance, what happens when you pump water into pipes? As water moves through pipes, it's forced into right angles. How does water flow in nature? It flows over rocks gently, side to side. This vortexing action, along with the natural electromagnetic properties of the Earth and minerals, create this "structured water." There's a rhythmic pattern to it. By forcing water into right angles, we destructure it from the natural shape it wants to take. That damage impacts the water in surprising ways, but the simplest is that the taste and feel completely change. Again, take the opportunity to drink water straight from the source, and you'll see immediately what I mean.

Let's nerd out a little on structured water. Structured water goes by many names: Coherent water, EZ water, hexagonal water, and ordered water, but all describe the same phenomenon. This type of water forms an ordered pattern when it's next to "hydrophilic" (water-loving) surfaces. You learn in third-grade science that water has three states: liquid, solid, and gas, but there is that fourth state, which is a gel-like substance called structured water. This gel makes up a majority of the cell's interior. Why do you think that blood doesn't pour out of you like a faucet when you cut yourself?

On top of the damage to the water the pipes cause, most municipally-sourced water for major cities has been treated with chlorine and other chemicals. These kill the bacteria and pathogens but also do further damage to the structure of the water. By the time you drink it, the water has stored a lot of negativity in its memory. You can think of this water as damaged. If water has memory, which I believe it does, then it remembers everything that has happened to it since the beginning of time. It's like storing computer information on magnetic tape. Could you imagine the profound implications if we could crack this code?

If you buy bottled water, even if it claims to be "pristine, protected, glacial run-off filtered through volcanic rocks for a minimum of ten thousand years" (I'm being facetious here, obviously), you run into a similar problem. These waters still remember their long commercial journey from the spring to the store. The good news is water is also incredibly resilient. When water is in its natural form in lakes, rivers, streams, etc. it has the ability to cleanse itself, ridding itself of the negative inputs and energies. Isn't nature f'kn amazing?

Experiments on Water

There have been many other experiments that prove the powerful memory of water. In one, scientists showed that water remembers what it has been subjected to. To prove this, they first measured the frequency of the water. Then, they put a leaf in the water and measured the frequency again. Finally, they removed the leaf and took one last measurement. This final snapshot was a mirror of the second. The impact of the leaf in the water was perfectly preserved.

Everything in the world is a vibration, and the water picks up on those vibrations. Any vibration has the potential to change the structure of water, no matter how small. That's why touch is so important—the water within your body knows if you've been touched, hugged, or kissed. Even your thoughts can change the structure of the water.

That's why praying over somebody can help them heal—we're all vibrations, and the water within them picks up on that positive energy and uses it to help heal them. Why do you think people pray over water or bathe in holy water? Or even bless their meals before they consume them? Water is likely consciousness, and the ancient people knew that.

As stated earlier, water responds uniquely to every individual. This may be a reason why it's hard to do empirical experiments with water. If water "doesn't like you," or you don't like yourself (hint hint, you are mostly water), are you going to get sick more often? Dr. Emoto's experiments make you wonder.

While some scientists are trying to figure out the behavior of water, some skeptics believe there's no such thing as information in water and water behaves the way they expect it to. This is a mystical relationship, and it doesn't fit into the narrow boundaries of logic and reason they've developed.

By the time water goes through all of that processing, treatment, and unnatural energy absorption, what do you think the water you're drinking is really like? Do you think it has the power to bring you life?

The Importance of Structured Water

Structured water retains its memory, which means it retains its ability to process and exchange information. When structured water interacts with cellular components such as proteins, they perform the functions they are designed to do. One of those functions is the proper folding of proteins to allow them to carry out various functions.

When a disproportionate amount of unstructured water in the cells exists, the proteins might misfold. When this happens on a chronic basis, it is probably causing cellular stress. Your body constantly needs to replenish this supply of water. If it enters the body already structured, it is theorized to cause less stress on the body.

The problem comes when you drink destructured water. Let me emphasize this again so it's crystal clear: destructured water is demineralized water as well as energetically polluted water. So just because you mineralize the water doesn't mean it hasn't stored a lot of negativity. This is where blessing, thanking, and loving your water starts your healing journey. Before it can be properly used, your body has to structure it for your use. That takes a huge amount of energy and resources. The more destructured water you drink, the more stress it can cause on the bodily systems. In fact, destructured water has lost some of its natural negative charge. For people who drink unstructured water, it is estimated that up to *fifty percent* of their daily energy is spent just reversing that charge so their bodies can use the water.

I'm not alone in these claims. Consider the quotes by Dr. Carly Nuday, Ph.D., in her book *Water Codes*:

> *Science can now show that the DNA in our bodies is literally encased in and surrounded by liquid water crystals that are structured in complex, sacred geometrical form...*
>
> *Unfortunately, it takes more energy for the body to restructure water than it receives from the*

water itself.

Since most of us are drinking exclusively destructured and demineralized water, we're wasting vast resources adapting it for our body's use. If we break that cycle and drink water directly in its purest form, we can start to transform our health. It improves digestion and sleep and reduces chronic inflammation and, most importantly, cellular oxidative stress. Again, it helps to improve all the cellular factors on the green side of the Ultimate Health Model™.

Is Alkaline Water Beneficial?

Understand that alkaline water is artificially made with electricity versus alkalinity, which is water that has minerals in it. The alkaline water might have benefits, but for extra assurance, add minerals to it such as Himalayan salt, Celtic salt, or sea salt as extra assurance.

Many people believe that cancer grows in an acidic environment. While studies show this is probably true, drinking alkaline water is not going to alkalize your body. , we now know that alkaline water is made using electricity that artificially pulls water molecules apart, creating a high pH synthetically with no actual minerals. Your body then depletes its own reserves trying to use something that isn't there because water is very aggressive and needs substances dissolved in it. Why do you think water is known as the universal solvent? And besides, wouldn't alkaline water, when it hits the stomach, become acidic?

Structured water has several other benefits:

1. It has a greater capacity to oxygenate the body.
2. It increases cell capacity for memory and information storage.
3. It transports minerals more efficiently.
4. It most likely is more efficient at carrying nutrients to the cell and taking away waste and toxins.
5. It provides an increased capacity to the cells for regulation, regeneration, and healing.
6. It acts as an antioxidant.

Let's look at the first point in more detail. Oxygen is critical for health. It has a negative charge, which increases the negative charge of the cell to regulate and heal. When the water is in these hexagonal-type shapes, they are theorized to hold more oxygen because of the charge ratios from the hydrogen and oxygen atoms. Cancer does not proliferate in a high-oxygen environment. As we discussed in the previous chapters, it thrives in more hypoxic (low oxygen) conditions because it ferments nutrients. That means that the more oxygenated your tissues and cells are, the less susceptible you are to disease. Tattoo this last statement on your other damn arm!

That's how important it is.

We have been talking a lot about structured water in this chapter, but understand that just drinking more water in general helps alleviate chronic conditions.

In the body, structured water acts as an antioxidant because of its increased ability to hold oxygen. This is crucial. We all have heard of antioxidants ad nauseam. But you probably had no idea that structured water is one of the most powerful antioxidants.

As the famous Indian doctor Batmanghelidj said, "You're not sick. You're just thirsty." Chronic dehydration, as our model states, is one of the contributing cellular factors to chronic disease. Did you know that high cholesterol levels are linked to dehydration? We will tackle these cholesterol myths in the next chapter.

The Structure of Fruits and Vegetables

This is a controversial opinion, but that's why you're reading this book, right? The reason I believe fruits and vegetables have some benefit *isn't* because of the miraculous benefits of phytochemicals or phytonutrients. These compounds are designed to protect the plants and are not essential for human health. In fact, some phytonutrients like polyphenols and flavonoids may be pro-oxidants and act as anti-nutrients in high amounts. They're good for you because they're a source of structured water. Period. The antioxidant in produce is the water! Produce is between eighty and ninety-five percent water. All whole foods contain structured water! That's the main reason they are healthy. What's not in processed food? Water! Are the pieces starting to fall into place?

Linus Pauling, an American chemist, famously said, "You can trace every sickness, every disease, and every ailment to a mineral deficiency." One of these major minerals is magnesium. Studies show that a large percentage of the population is deficient in magnesium. This has been linked to cardiovascular problems because magnesium is needed to keep the calcium in the bones and teeth and not the arteries, which can lead to calcification.

That's why drinking natural spring water is beneficial: it has the perfect balance of minerals, including magnesium. The minerals are like a scaffolding that water uses to structure itself to create and store information. When you drink demineralized water—as an example, consider reverse osmosis—it causes stress on the cells because of the lack of minerals.

A quick search on the internet shows multiple theories and claims about how water gets into cells. The truth is, nobody knows for sure. My hypothesis is the body's cells have what's called an aquaporin channel, the plumbing system of the cell that helps facilitate water molecule transport. It is one of the ways cells regulate their water. When you drink structured water, it enters cells more efficiently. When water is destructured, water forms larger clusters that make it more difficult to enter cells, as they have to be broken down to facilitate proper cell nourishment. The body has to break down the clusters into smaller clusters to be able to be absorbed into these aquaporin channels. Water can also diffuse through the cell membrane because of its extremely small size.

Structured water can also transmute toxins. For example, glyphosate is made of a combination of phosphorus, nitrogen, hydrogen, oxygen, and carbon atoms. Together, they may become toxic, but their toxicity levels are reduced when broken down into elemental forms. There are experts who disagree, but I believe it is plausible for structured water to have these abilities to "detoxify" and break down substances because, as discussed earlier, water acts like a liquid crystal.

As you age, you lose the capacity to sustain the energy of this action to constantly structure water. You dehydrate even though you have water in your body because of our model. And if your body is confronted with diseases or illnesses, it has a more difficult time in the healing process.

That's why the third important power of structured water is the energy it brings you. The first thing you should do to mitigate a chronic condition is start a regiment of drinking structured water. Try it. It can't harm you, only benefit you. That way, the body can stop wasting energy restructuring water and use its energies for healing and rebuilding.

EMFs Disrupt Structured Water

EMFs are all around us. Whether it's your phone, your computer, or other electronics, they give off radiation. That energy disrupts the structure of the water in your body, causing chronic inflammation as well as the other negative cellular factors in our model. Numerous studies implicate the damage from EMFs. Disease is a combination of all the negative lifestyle factors in the model, but EMFs might be the icing on the cake. I will talk more about electromagnetic frequencies (EMFs) in Chapter 9.

Together, all of these factors make structured water one of the most important facets to reclaiming your health.

How to Find Structured Water

The best way to get structured water is directly from a spring. These are free to access. You can collect the spring water in large jugs, and you want to store it in a cool dark place. This will inhibit growth of algae. (Side note: Some research suggests that green algae might be cancer protective. Why do you think people take spirulina as a supplement? It's a form of algae. See "Health Benefits of Blue Green Algae: Prevention of Cardivascular Disease and Non Alcohlic Fatty Liver Disease" in the Journal of Medicinal Food, 2013, 16(2) 103-1110). If you decide to utilize a spring, make sure to have the water tested before you drink it. Some springs may have human contaminants like pesticides or arsenic.

Another option if you don't live near a spring or don't own a car to transport the water, is to invest in a machine like a water vortexer. I strongly suggest devices from MEA Water Company and use them myself. Water vortex machines swirl the water and artificially recreate the conditions that create structured water in nature. Visit the Recommendations page on my website to find resources.

Unfortunately, these machines won't physically infuse the water with the minerals you need if it's already been processed, but they can restructure water that's experienced trauma or destructuring on its commercial path. Therefore, it *energetically* infuses the water by structuring it. You can add Himalayan salt or natural sea salt to water, as these have a balance of minerals in them. A caution on the sea salt: most of our oceans have been polluted with plastics and trash. These microplastics can be in some sea salts. So, find a salt source you trust.

Cosmic towers are extremely expensive but are worth mentioning. They work slightly differently by building up their own supply of pure life-force energy, benefiting any living organism in its field. They increase the body's production of electrons and prevent the destruction of the hexagonal water structures of our body caused by EMFs.

Another strategy to improve your water is to write on your glasses or water bottles and tell the water that you love it. *Anything* you can do to appreciate, love, nurture, and respect the water is your goal. Funny? Well, when you start respecting water, you start respecting yourself.

I know some people might say it's mumbo jumbo. They might even call it pseudoscience. Well, they can say what they want. I've seen the power of structured water firsthand. I've watched the impact on my health, and I can't wait for you to experience the same health benefits I have found for myself.

WHY ARE YOU SICK?

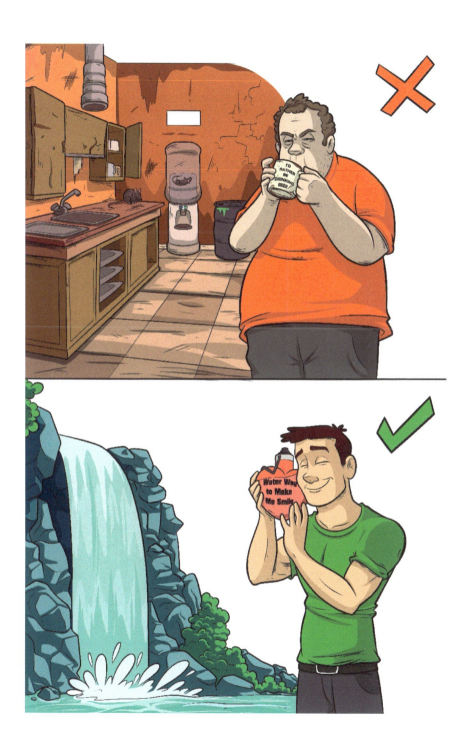

If there is magic on this planet, it is contained in water.
~Loren Eiseley

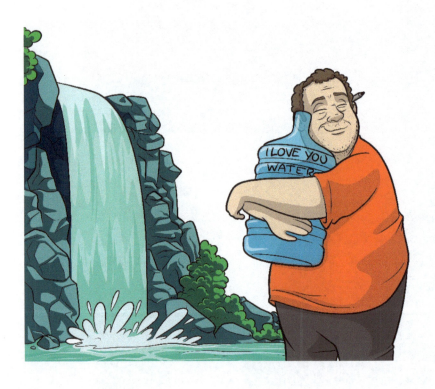

CHAPTER 7
Food

Everything comes from the soil, including our food. If we continue to destroy the soil, the result could be catastrophic.
~ Benjamin Smith

I'm quoting myself above, and let me expand. Understand this: the more we deplete the soil, the sicker the population will become, PERIOD! Industrial agriculture, monocropping (growing the same crop one year after year without soil rest and biodiversity), improper management of grazing animals, and general poor farming practices are all hurting the soil. More about that ahead.

In the meantime, a proper diet is real food. That's it. Anything that God put on this earth to eat is a whole food. Anything else, don't eat it. A proper diet is an authentic, one-ingredient whole food. Don't eat sugar or processed foods. Ultra-processed foods cause stress on the mitochondria. There are no micronutrients in ultra-processed foods. Even when stuff is added, like sprayed-on synthetic vitamins to fortify cereals, your body does not know how to process that. Your body does not process anything in a box or bag, especially with unpronounceable ingredients, in the same way.

Build Up the Body

When I first started this journey, I was like everybody else. My relationship with food was completely out of whack.

I was a really skinny kid, and as a child, I was teased a lot. No matter how much I ate, it seemed like I never put on weight. I never had a girlfriend, and I was shy and self-conscious all the time.

When I turned eighteen, I decided that if I couldn't put on weight, I would put on muscle. *If I get big, I'll finally be happy*, I thought. I started working out a lot and eating a ton of food to help build my body up. I still had trouble keeping on the weight, so I started eating huge amounts of protein powders and carb-heavy foods. I ate six or seven times a day, making sure my blood sugar never went down.

I lived in constant terror of losing weight. If I missed a single meal, I got a horrible headache, and felt "hangry." My favorite catchphrase was "I gotta eat!" When that happened, carbs were my only rescue.

One day, when I was in my early thirties, I went to see my sister. The timing of the trip was awkward, and I had to miss a few meals. I didn't eat for about eight hours, and as I sat there in her living room, waiting for dinner, I started to stutter. It had never happened before, and it absolutely freaked me out. I couldn't control my mouth or my words.

"What the h-h-hell is g-g-going on?" I gasped.

"Oh, you're fine," my sister said. "You just need dinner. Don't worry about it."

Well, I did worry. When I got home, I immediately went to see the doctor. "Oh, you're fine," the doctor said. "You're in great shape. Just keep your blood sugar up."

I knew the doctor was wrong, and I was petrified. I didn't know then what I know now about inflammation or the dangers of sugar. I just knew I never wanted to stutter like that again. I decided to give up on my bodybuilding and high-carb diet and try a low-carb diet. *We didn't have access to many carbs in my ancestors' days*, I figured. *My body makes its own sugar, so I don't see why I should be eating any of it.*

I was scared of losing weight or of feeling hungry, but I was also scared of the lack of control I had over my body. It was time to make a change.

A low-carb diet allows approximately one hundred daily grams of carbs. That's two small servings a day—say, hash browns in the morning and a cup of rice at dinner. Keto, as a comparison, allows approximately fifty grams of carbs or fewer a day, while people who don't watch their carbs can easily consume around three hundred daily grams.

For the first two weeks, I felt horrible. I almost gave up a hundred times. "I'm not going to do this. This is too hard. I'm hungry. I need to eat." This is why people fail, but I stuck with it. You have to fight through it.

Then, something magical happened. Around the third or fourth week, my hunger completely vanished. My stutter went away. I stopped getting headaches, and I stopped feeling stressed about my weight, which stayed stable. I ate more meat and more meat, and I felt better and better. The little aches and pains I experienced for years vanished. I could skip a meal—or two, or three—and not feel hungry.

All because I was giving my body what it actually needed. For the first time, I was listening to it instead of my fear, and the results were transformational.

I tell this story because it is the textbook example of people addicted to carbs. If I could sum up this chapter in one sentence it would be this: eat one-ingredient whole foods that were put here by Mother Nature. That's it! This topic has been convoluted, confused, and complicated on purpose. With this understanding alone, your decision-making will be freed up tremendously.

The Importance of Food

When you understand that food is information, you can either put good information into your body or bad information. Why is food information? As we discussed in the last chapter, it is because food is comprised mostly of water, specifically structured water. Interestingly, your body's preferred source of fuel is water. I'm not talking about the water bound to nutrients, but the free water you consume. It is considered clean energy because there are no byproducts of waste. What's not needed is excreted as urine. On the other hand, food, especially refined carbs, are dirty fuel, as their byproducts are fat storage, which has its own metabolic risks.

All right, are you ready to geek out again? Water is the body's, and in particular the brain's, preferred energy source because specialized receptors on the cell membranes, along with minerals, spin these receptors with the rushing flow of water. This produces ATP (the energy currency of the cell and electricity). Hmmm . . . What is the analogy to man's creation? A hydroelectric power plant. Mind-blown! Another reason to stay hydrated.

If you choose good information, you also choose to reclaim better health. Conversely, if you choose bad information (ultra-processed foods, vegetable oils, refined sugars, and flours) or foods devoid of water, you are likely on the road to poor health.

Knowing the importance of food helps you pay more attention to the *kind* of foods you eat, as well as the category of food that you eat. You think about its origins and how it impacts your overall health. You find a greater understanding of what food means to you, and you start to reclaim your health.

When you just blindly consume food without any awareness, you are potentially putting your body in a state of stress—especially the mitochondria. Without awareness, you lose control of your vitality and are enslaved to food companies. If you want to live on the red side, then thank the food companies for your meals. Ultra-processed foods are keeping you satisfied and not hungry. I you want to live on the green side, then you'll choose healthier options. It really is your choice.

Food is a living thing. It has energy and, thanks to the structured water within it, also stores information. You process all of those stored memories and energy every time you eat. It's no wonder food is such a huge contributor to our health. The food you eat should be infused with as much positive energy as possible.

When you eat fresh fruits and vegetables from your own garden, the love you put into growing that food comes back to you. The same is true when you eat meat from a small farm or buy eggs from someone who cares for their chickens. According to Dr. Sarah Pugh, a quantum biologist and researcher, you're telling your mitochondria where you are in time and space when you eat locally and seasonally. I know that sounds far-fetched, but it all has to do with energy.

The problem is we have a global economy where all food is available 24/7. Why is this a problem? Our ancient ancestors had to eat what was in season, which was a few wild berries, some nuts or seeds they could forage, or some wild cabbage they could munch on. Ready for another shocking fact? The leafy greens and cruciferous vegetables all have a common ancestor! That's wild cabbage! They've been hybridized and bred into existence. How could broccoli and arugula be essential if they have only been around for approximately the last 5,000 years? I guess the mantra "Eat the rainbow" would have puzzled Joe Caveman!

Looking Local

I get eggs from a local farm. I've talked to the woman who runs it, and I asked her, "How do you take care of your chickens?"

"Oh, we love our chickens," she told us. "We hand

feed them, and we let them run around the pasture and get lots of exercise. They all have names and personalities, and we know them."

Those eggs are the most delicious I've ever had. You can taste the love and freedom with every bite. You have to connect to your food, whether it's a side of beef or the microbes in your garden's soil, which are key players in making plants grow.

When you buy food from huge, impersonal corporations, you are very likely buying produce grown in soil that is severely deficient in minerals. Why? Because they spray pesticides that kill the soil. As a result, the soil is depleted of nutrients and essential microbes, one of the key players in our ecosystem. The organisms (or microbes) produce certain acids (called humic and fulvic acids), which provide the plants with much of their nutrition. These acids are able to break down the minerals in the soil and make them bioavailable to the plants. They also help transport and contribute to the plant's overall health.

Now, we are going off to left field. I want you to visualize the microbes as miniature people. The soil is their home. The ground cover and plants are their "roofs." When we use pesticides and chemicals, those are "bombs." When the soil is tilled and plowed, we are destroying the roofs. Why do you think bare soil dries out? Most likely, you have heard of the Dust Bowl of the 1930s. If you haven't, this is an event that happened in the Midwest. Years of poor soil management and damaging destructive agricultural practices caused the soil to turn into dust. Without adequate irrigation back then, the farmers couldn't maintain the soil. Consequently, huge dust storms engulfed the Midwest.

We need to respect the soil, just like my quote says. If you own grazing land, one important and all-natural way to improve it is to keep cows or other ruminants on your property (goat, sheep, deer, buffalo, etc.). Cows are natural lawnmowers and chew the grass down to a beneficial height that stimulates growth. When grasses are too tall, the photosynthesis is impeded. When grasses are too short, the photosynthesis is also impeded. When farmers implement rotational grazing, photosynthesis is improved.

Note also that cow manure is one of the most beneficial additives you can use to replenish the soil, as Mother Nature intended, instead of the terrible fertilizers some farmers use today. Microbes deeply connect to the topic of soil. Plants take carbon dioxide out of the air and turn it into carbohydrates that the soil microbes feed on, including carbonic acid (carbon metabolites). Soil microbes also feed on nitrogen nitrate metabolites through the roots and into the soil. It's a symbiotic relationship.

What's one of the big topics being preached today? Climate change. Well, I've got news for you. It's not only the cows belching and farting or the massive consumption of fossil fuels causing it. It's also the destruction of our soils. Those cute little microbes we talked about earlier actually sequester a large portion of carbon. Healthy soil is a huge carbon sink. This is one of the factors of climate change that's being quietly swept under the rug. And don't think your environmentally-conscious electric car is doing the planet any favors. Most electricity is made from fossil fuels. Brake dust from vehicles contributes more particulate matter to the atmosphere than exhaust fumes. *What?* Damn! And I thought I was helping to save the planet.

Before I get off of my soapbox, please understand how important soil health is to the future of our planet. It's not just about cutting emissions; it's about removing the excess carbon and other greenhouse gases from the atmosphere. Here is a really scary analogy about how much carbon is actually in the air. Every time the CO_2 concentration goes up by approximately 1% in the atmosphere, there is an equivalent amount of carbon contained in solid form at approximately 2.1 billion tons or a brick of carbon a kilometer long and a kilometer thick! For a graphical representation of this, do an online search for Ayres Rock in Australia. You bet your ass people would pay attention to that if it was floating over your city!

Do you see a correlation here? Sick soil equals sick plants equals sick humans. Some studies show that a person needs to consume approximately ten apples today to get the same mineral content they got from a single apple fifty years ago. I guess these pesticides damage the environment as well as your health.

Or what about a chicken kept in a cage, never seeing sunlight, and fed artificial GMO grains? It's going to be deficient in vitamin D, which means you are eating deficient chicken. Be aware that many feedlot cows are fed antibiotics and hormones to make them get bigger and fatter so they can be slaughtered sooner—and you gobble up those hormones with every bite. I hope this makes you think about what you're eating.

If you care about your food, you care about yourself.

The Cost of Good Health

A lot of people hesitate to buy healthier food because of the cost. The truth is, though, that you can take the time to shop around and get good deals from local farmers, just like you can at big supermarket chains. At least do some research and see what's out there. Advocate for yourself. If you're located within a "food desert," consider planting herbs and produce on your windowsills, patio, or backyard. Plus, you have to consider the cost of health care. Do you want to pay a little more for healthy food now, or a whole lot at the doctor when you get sick from putting poison in your body? Either way, you end up paying.

Let's look at some of the foods we've been trained to eat that are really unhealthy—sugar, seed oils, and grains—as well as one thing that's healthier than you've been led to believe.

A Note on Studies

Before we dive into the evil three, I want to revisit the topic of nutritional studies—and why they seem to constantly contradict each other.

On Monday, you read that red meat causes cancer. But on Tuesday, you read that red meat increases your life expectancy. On Thursday, you read that butter is associated with heart disease. By Friday, a new article says, "Saturated fat does not cause heart disease."

As a consumer, what are you supposed to do? How are you supposed to eat anything?

Let's say you see an article from *a medical journal*. That's a trustworthy source, right? The headline reads, "Study shows that red meat is associated with a 20 percent increase in cancer." Sounds scary . . . but is it really?

For example, the narrative that meat causes cancer doesn't even pass the cursory test for common sense.

We have been eating it for a million years, and suddenly it causes disease? Moreover, meat consumption has steadily declined over the past 50 years, yet chronic disease rates are rising. You know from my diagram and model what the true underlying factors are that contribute to disease. And cholesterol, saturated fat, and meat aren't on there!

What that headline actually means is that the scientists and researchers have sent out questionnaires asking people what they ate. This is called an observational study and relies on people's memories. After all, people who journal what they eat, especially days or weeks later, are notoriously inaccurate about what they report. Then the researchers tabulate the results and say, "All of these people have cancer, and they all ate red meat. Therefore, red meat causes cancer."

Even many so-called "random control trials" are inaccurate and invalid. It's a misnomer because there are a gazillion co-factors that aren't taken into account. They can't control factors that are uncontrollable by definition, like stress, and therefore cannot determine cause and effect. Therefore, scientists say the results are "associated," which is a broad generalized hypothesis.

For instance, we may be "shown" that there's a connection or association between eating red meat and getting cancer… or a *correlation*. It does *not* prove that eating red meat *causes* cancer. Nothing in nutritional science is causal. Hundreds of confounding factors have to be taken into consideration by the researchers. For instance, maybe wealthy people can afford to eat more red meat. Furthermore, what are these people eating with the red meat? Are they drinking soda? Eating French fries? What about the hamburger buns and pasta they are wolfing down in unbelievable quantities?

Or what about the other factors we have already discussed in previous chapters? How much inflammation do people have? How about their sleeping or breathing habits? Do you see why nutritional studies are often invalid? Yet, policies and guidelines are built on these skewed reports.

All nutritional studies are based on *correlation*, not *causation*.

Scientists and industry-funded studies also contribute to bias. Believe it or not, these epidemiologists (the term for this type of science) actually lie. They use terms like "adjusted for confounders," which means they fudge the results to get the outcome they want. When I first learned how nutritional studies were conducted, I was like, *WTF?* I've been lied to and bamboozled. How can this even be legal? So now that you're armed with this information, they could say something as ridiculous as "Eggs cause suicidal thoughts," and you can laugh!

I put a lot of stock in science. But there's just no way to be accurate on nutritional studies, which is why you have to base your decisions on the science we *do* know and understand. That's why I talk a lot about how the body works and the processes that happen inside of you when you eat certain foods—foods like the evil three. Before we discuss the "triad of demise," let's dispel a few myths about calories.

A calorie is a calorie: This couldn't be farther from the truth. Are you telling me that a hundred calories worth of soda or chocolate is the same as a hundred calories worth of meat or vegetables? Does this even make common damn sense? One food has water, minerals, vitamins, and nutrients. And soda? It is metabolized in completely different ways within the body. It's not rocket science.

Calories in / calories out: This one has been ingrained in the proverbial "public mind" since we started counting them. Calories are a measure of heat generated by a sample in a bomb calorimeter. That's it. It has nothing to do with how this energy is converted into chemical energy in the body. Furthermore, with inflammation, stress, dehydration, and all the cellular circles, it is impossible to know how many "calories" you're consuming, absorbing, or excreting, for that matter. Did our ancestors count calories? *No*. This ties into why diets don't work long-term. You can't starve your body and expect no ramifications. Not to mention, you can only "white knuckle it" so long. You need to change your eating habits for the rest of your life, and these "evil three"—refined sugar, refined grains/carbs, and seed oils—are getting in the way.

Snacking: Although mainstream culture has convinced us that snacking is okay, this couldn't be farther from the truth. We are not cows. We are not designed to graze all day. Why? Every time you put anything in your mouth other than water or pure fat (gross), you illicit an insulin response. I don't care if it is a glass of orange juice or a stale candy bar you find hidden in a glove box and eat because you're "hangry." Chronically elevated insulin levels are damaging to your health. This is well documented.

The Evil Three

If you are going to cut just three things out of your diet, it should be the evil three: refined sugar, refined grains, and seed oils. Let's look at each in more detail.

Refined sugar: We all know how great it tastes, but sugar is terrible for your body. It can lead to all of the five circles on the red side of our model and, in turn, contributes to every chronic disease. Let me emphasize that we are talking about refined sugars, not moderate amounts of fruit sugars.

Where it gets complicated is that fructose, glucose, and galactose are all forms of sugar. The table sugar we all know and love is called sucrose. It's half glucose and half fructose. When you eat something with any of these sugars, even so-called "healthy grains" (which are starch-based), your body will convert it to blood sugar. A lot of people think avoiding sugar just means avoiding sweets. What they don't understand is that all of those carbohydrates are being converted into sugar, and that does more damage than a hit straight from the sugar cane because of nature's sugar regulation system: **fiber**.

You might be asking yourself, *I thought grains have fiber?* This is correct if you are consuming "whole grains" since they do contain small amounts of fiber. But I believe the damaging effects of the sugar, not to mention anti-nutrients in grains, offset its benefits.

Why are refined sugar and refined carbs so bad? Let's make an analogy to cooking. Why do cooks add sugar to water in recipes? To thicken it. Your blood is mostly water, approximately eighty percent. Do you see a problem here? If the blood gets too thick, it impedes flow. That's why your body has to remove sugar from circulation as quickly as possible with the help of the hormone insulin. Let's elaborate a little more on the insulin-sugar connection. The medical establishment focuses on controlling blood glucose. As long as your blood glucose levels are in the normal range, then everything is fine. Wrong. News flash! The body has to keep your blood sugar in check; otherwise, you die. It's the insulin doing that.

Once your blood sugar goes out of control, it is called type 2 diabetes.

Unfortunately, your insulin has been elevated for decades. Finally, it gives up trying to control blood sugar and says, F*** it! This is why insulin levels are a way better predictor of your health, not blood sugar. The good news is that fiber in fruit and vegetables slows this onslaught of sugar into your body and cells.

By now, you're wondering what else you have been lied to about. Just wait! There's plenty more.

A quick word about fructose. This sugar, according to Dr. Robert Lustig, a pediatric endocrinologist at the University of California, San Francisco, specializing in childhood obesity, says that fructose is exponentially more detrimental than glucose. Why? Because the liver is the only way for your body to process fructose. When you overwhelm it, you are contributing to nonalcoholic fatty liver disease (NAFL). What the liver can't process is turned into fat. Why do you think there's an epidemic of NAFL?

Another interesting fact about fat is that you have three depots of fat storage: subcutaneous (under the skin), visceral (around your organs), and liver. The liver fat is the most damaging. This fat is the most metabolically active, meaning it secretes inflammatory chemicals that harm your body. Suffice it to say that your liver can only deal with approximately a half pound extra of fat. That's it. Just because you're thin doesn't mean you are healthy.

High fructose corn syrup or foods in which the fiber has been stripped away are like an injection—or instant shock—to the system. If you eat a lot of fructose, you overwhelm the liver. Fructose is stored as fat in the liver and muscle cells and can cause fatty liver disease.

However, your body processes fruits more easily because the fiber in fruit slows the onslaught of fructose into the liver. For instance, a piece of fruit might have five grams of fructose compared to soft drinks that can have upwards of fifty grams.

You've been told your whole life that fruit juices are good, but there is no fiber to slow the onslaught of a sugar rush. If you are eating a whole food diet, you can include a little bit of fruit and a bit of organic honey, but not too much. Again, we don't want to overwhelm the liver and trigger fatty liver disease or any other potential chronic condition.

Newsflash: orange juice isn't doing you any favors because the vitamin C you are "supposedly" getting is competing with the sugar to get into your cells. Sugar wins out every time.

"But My Body Needs Sugar!"

Our bodies need sugar to function, but many people

mistakenly believe that means we need to eat at least a small amount of sugar in order to be healthy. The truth is that your body can make its own sugar from non-sugar sources. It's called gluconeogenesis. You don't need a single gram of carbohydrates or sugar in your diet, ever. If you don't eat any protein or any fat, you will likely die. But sugar and carbs? They're extraneous.

Grains: The second evil is grains or refined carbs. You may think you're being healthy by eating whole wheat or twelve-grain bread instead of white, but your body is turning it all to sugar. It contributes to inflammation, and it also contributes to problems in your gut, like leaky gut. Your only saving grace is that it contains some fiber, which, as we now know, slows the absorption. My theory, backed by other scientists, suggests that many of our ancient ancestors didn't eat an abundance of grains. So why do we think we can eat them now?

Consider the "Egyptian Mummy Diet." The ancient Egyptians based their diet mostly on grains (not good). I don't care if the grains were grown on land blessed by a priest! Interestingly, *NPR* published a report on July 26, 2016, titled "Mummified Egyptian Was Just As Sedentary And Carb-Hungry As Modern Men." Autopsies on mummies have revealed surprising atherosclerotic plaques (or the beginnings of heart disease). The effect of these grains can also be evidenced in the statues and figurines they left behind, which have big bellies and "man boobs." Some critics will say that it was the meat in their diets that caused this because the only people who were mummified were the wealthy. I disagree. The wealthy ate just as much bread as the impoverished.

I theorize, most likely, that the reason they were unhealthy-looking was because of the chronic activation of the Randle cycle we discussed earlier. As discussed, carbs and fat together in excess cause inflammation. It's that simple.

Some people may argue it's just the refined and processed grains that are hard on your health. I have bad news for you: it isn't. All grains are bad when they are transformed into flour. Why? Because this instantly raises blood sugar and causes inflammation. This is the same problem with refined sugar. Very little redeeming nutritional value exists in refined grains, although suffice it to say that whole grains have a little more nutritional value due to fiber.

Let me reiterate that the microbes in the gut produce short-chain fatty acids (saturated fats) when they feed on fiber. You have two choices when it comes to the microbiome in the gut, where the plant material is fermenting: 1.) animal-based diet or a 2.) plant-based diet. Pick one, and stay in your lane or you're going to crash. No weaving or swerving. Remember the Randle cycle?

Let's consider the Carnivore Diet. The microbes in the gut must be feeding on something besides fiber. Right? Studies show that protein can be used as a fuel source for microbes as well as ketone bodies made from fat because you're not eating carbs. As you know, the typical American diet consists of ultra-processed foods—not whole foods like fruits, veggies, and animal products. The typical Western diet consists of refined crap, and there is nothing available for the microbes to feed on because you aren't giving them what they need. So what do the microbes feed on in this case? The answer is mucus (epithelial cells) in the intestine. This potentially contributes to leaky gut, autoimmune conditions, inflammation, and any chronic condition. In other words, the microbes feed on you. I'll repeat again and again because you need to remember this. It will help relieve that nagging pain in your gut.

When you eat grains, the gluten proteins make it difficult for the microbiome in your gut to break down, which may cause inflammation. This, in turn, pulls apart the zonulin proteins that hold the epithelial cells in the gut lining together. You're literally pulling apart the intestinal lining every time you eat grains.

That lets undigested food particles leak through the gut lining into your bloodstream and may contribute to autoimmune diseases, among other problems. We have all heard the terms gluten sensitivity and celiac disease. Gluten is just one antinutrient in plants—a naturally occurring substance that interferes with the absorption of nutrients. Oxalates, tannins, and phytic acids are others. I believe we are meant to eat plants in limited amounts for these reasons.

Seed oils: Canola oil. Sunflower oil. Safflower oil. Corn oil. The list goes on. Seed oils are in most of the ultra-processed foods found on store shelves, restaurants, school cafeterias, and our kitchens at home, too. The average American coats 30 percent of everything they eat in one seed oil or another. These oils weren't around one hundred years ago. Heart disease rates and chronic disease were also significantly lower a century ago. Several studies show a direct relationship between seed oil consumption and rising disease rates over that time.

Do you really understand how bad seed oils are for you, though? Well, after reading the next paragraph, I bet you run downstairs and toss that jar—or jug—of oil.

There is only a very minimal amount of oil in seeds. So seeds are pressed, heated, and then processed with solvents like hexane to turn them into seed oil. That oxidizes the oil further, and by now, you know how dangerous oxidation is for us. It causes inflammation, cellular stress, and dehydration. A good analogy for oxidation is what happens to metal when it oxidizes: it rusts. This is similar to seed oil consumption—except the worry is rancidity (rather than rust). That's what's happening internally when you consume seed oils. You are actually rusting from the inside out, or rather, consuming rancid oil.

Furthermore, these oils are washed and deodorized with sodium hydroxide. Do you know what that is in unscientific terms? Drain cleaner, which I personally don't want to be ingesting. Then it's deodorized with more bad stuff. Although the makers say that when the oil gets to the bottle, all these residues are gone, you should think twice. This probably leads to poor health, weight gain, and other diseases.

Seed oils are "unsaturated fats." Unsaturated fats have a molecular configuration that enables them to react more easily with oxygen, potentially causing oxidation (that you don't want). If you have to use oil in your cooking, options exist that are better for you. Olive oil, coconut oil, and avocado oil come from fruit, so they aren't processed like seed oils. But they might still be pressed or heated, which can diminish their nutritional value. Still, by definition of being unsaturated, there is still potential for oxidation.

You really want to look for *saturated* fat alternatives. Saturated fats are good for us:

- Butter

- Ghee
- Lard
- Bacon grease

The authorities will say, "No, those cause heart disease because they're saturated fat." Saturated fat isn't your enemy, and I hope the following will help you release your fear of fat.

Cholesterol and Saturated Fat

Saturated fats are essential for life! They are the components of hormones and cell membranes (think cell signaling and cell function) and serve as an energy source. Our bodies aren't as stupid as we are. If we don't want to eat fat, our bodies make fat from excess carbohydrates and proteins. One fat that is made from excess carbs is palmitic acid (saturated)!

Funny, earlier we mentioned that fiber is fermented into saturated fats. Yes, cows eat a saturated fat diet. Hmm?

For fifty years, we've been saying that saturated fat is bad because it raises the LDL cholesterol in your blood, and that's the "bad" cholesterol. HDL is the "good" cholesterol, and these are the parameters the medical community has been using since they discovered cholesterol. Let's define LDL and HDL before going further. LDL means low-density lipoprotein, and HDL is high-density lipoprotein. Since blood is mostly water and cholesterol is a waxy fat-like substance, these two things don't mix well! So nature invented an ingenious mechanism to transport this in particles called lipoproteins.

Here's another head-scratcher. Plants and all living things make cholesterol. Plant sterols are virtually identical to animal cholesterol. The truth is, though, that there's no such thing as good or bad cholesterol. Cholesterol measurements are just a snapshot in time—not static. It can change hourly, weekly, etc.

So if cholesterol "causes" vascular problems, do plants have vascular problems? Makes you think, huh? It's all about the way the cholesterol is carried in the bloodstream. Most tests measure the total amount of cholesterol in particles, which is, frankly, a useless measurement. LDL is not cholesterol. It is like a bus carrying cholesterol, vitamins, and fatty acids around the body, delivering vital nutrients to the cells. More about this a few paragraphs down.

In the 1950s, Ancel Keys, a nutritionist, did a huge study across seven countries to examine the effects of saturated fat on heart disease risk. He found that the more saturated fat, the more heart disease there was. It was a linear relationship, with the U.S. at the top on the far-right side and Japan at the bottom on the other side. The establishment bought into his study—hook, line, and sinker.

However, some people today believe that Keys omitted countries that didn't fit his correlation. The study is now highly contested. I think the dude lied and affected millions of lives!

And new evidence shows that cholesterol could be more important to our bodies than anyone wants to admit. Cholesterol makes up approximately fifty percent of your cell membranes. If you don't eat enough of it, your body makes it for you, up to three thousand milligrams a day. Question: How could something vital for life also be so detrimental? This is another WTF moment. While you're sitting there in your armchair reading this, think about that.

Cholesterol is also a precursor to your hormones. Testosterone, estrogen, and even cortisol start with cholesterol, and so does vitamin D. It should be called hormone D because it's made from cholesterol and acts as a hormone. Cholesterol is also the main ingredient in the myelin sheaths in your brain, which protect your nerves. Can you picture an electrical wire covered in rubber? The wire is your nerves, and the rubber is cholesterol in the form of a myelin sheath. Could this be why cholesterol-lowering medications have possible side effects such as impaired cognition?

Critics say that LDL is a risk factor for heart disease. The problem is that they are oversimplifying the issue. Chronic inflammation most likely causes heart disease, and this is not disputed. Cardiologists will say that inflammation is definitely a contributing factor to heart disease, but they don't agree about this initial cause.

Speaking of heart disease, do you know what that artery-blocking goop is made of? Well, it's not what you think. A very small percentage is made of cholesterol. And some of the cholesterol is actually plant sterols. Plants make a molecule almost identical to animal-based cholesterol. This has been found in the "plaques" (artery goop). These plaques also contain immune cells, red blood cell fragments (indicating a clotting process), and calcium. The calcium is laid down to protect the plaque from rupturing. Kinda like adding scar tissue. Oops! I guess plants don't have a free pass, especially refined flour and sugar.

Guess what? LDL is your friend. Look what the LDL cholesterol particles do below:

- Aids in fighting pathogens in your body by acting as an endogenous antioxidant.

- Is vitally important in transporting CoQ10 to the cells. CoQ10 is a powerful antioxidant protecting LDL and cell membranes. Think of this molecule as a spark plug that helps create energy in the mitochondria.

- Prevents calcification of the vascular system by converting vitamin K1 to vitamin K2 (K2 puts calcium where it's supposed be, like your teeth and bones and NOT your blood vessels).

When you know all of those facts, common sense prevails to tell you that LDL is good for us. We don't need a disputed study from the 1950s to make that decision.

More About Saturated Fats

Both saturated and unsaturated fats are found in each of your cell membranes. Most people believe that saturated fat clogs up the arteries like a pipe. That's just not true. Fat has to be transported in these particles because fat and water don't mix in the blood. It's transported in the LDL or HDL particles.

Which type of fat is better for the body? Saturated or unsaturated?

Do you know that saturated fat is less prone to oxidation than unsaturated fats? It has to do with its molecular configuration. "Saturated" means the fat molecule has no available site where oxygen can interact with it, whereas "unsaturated" means oxygen can interact with the fat molecule in one or more spots. On top of that, unsaturated fats are bent and curved, making them less stable than straight-shaped saturated fats.

Both are essential. Understand that if you don't eat saturated fat, your body will make it from fiber, or it will take sugar after it's been processed in the liver and convert it to fat, saturated or unsaturated, according to what the body needs.

The dogma that LDL causes heart disease is too simplistic. In reality, when the LDL particles are damaged due to glycation or oxidation (both cause inflammation), that creates a cascade of steps that lead to possible damage to the blood vessels. Do you see once again how the red cellular factors on the model initiate this? We have all been brainwashed into thinking cholesterol is bad, but that just doesn't make sense.

Eating carbs and fat together triggers the Randle cycle, which we discussed in Chapter 3. In that case, and only in that case, fat can potentially be bad for you. But if you're avoiding excess refined carbs, like you hopefully will be after reading this chapter, you don't have to worry about constantly activating the Randle cycle.

What *Should* You Eat?

It may be hard to hear, but this is the simple truth: a high-carb, high-sugar diet produces free radicals in your cells. Antioxidants help to mop up that pollution, but you're better off not making it in the first place. Do not follow a high-sugar ultra-processed food diet, which produces free radicals in the cells. *Voila*—inflammation, just like the model says. I'm a genius, agreed? Ha ha ha!

A lot of people think, *I can't eat that much protein! It's going to cause gout! The uric acid build-up causes uric acid crystals!* Don't worry. You won't get gout if you don't have the chronic inflammation produced by a poor diet and the other red lifestyle factors on the Ultimate Health Model™. I also hear the ridiculous phrase, "It's hard on the kidneys." Bullshit. I've been on this diet for years, and I've never been healthier. I even got a coronary artery calcium scan. It measures calcium buildup in your arteries. One of the factors in people who have heart attacks is blockages in their arteries. I wanted to make sure mine were healthy.

I got a score of zero. No buildup at all.

If you start to feel sick in the first month of your new diet, don't worry. When you eat a low-carb diet, your body has to rebuild the proteins and molecules that have been dormant in your high-carb lifestyle to become metabolically flexible, and you can burn both fat and carbs. But it takes time for that process of gut microbiome conversion. While your body is making that change, it often results in what's called keto flu.

The older you get, the worse the process feels because you have more inflammation and every other factor on the red side of the Ultimate Health Model™—more stress and more dehydration to fight against. But if you can fight through it, you'll be amazed at how great you feel when your body adjusts.

Here are a few more important rules to remember if you want to get a healthy diet.

Eat for water content: Fruits and vegetables are about ninety percent water. Meat and eggs are about sixty percent. You better be sitting down for this next sentence because it will blow your mind (good news). Besides the water content of eggs (a superfood with minerals, essential fatty acid, and all the nutrients you need for life), the oval shape is nature's water structuring device. This water is constantly structuring because of the flow pattern of the liquid in the egg. Remember, students, that we talked about structured water in Chapter 6 (the Water Chapter). Eggs are the most perfect food you could possibly eat.

Meanwhile, grains and ultra-processed foods have very little water content. Water is the most important thing on the planet for your health. If you eat a fresh fruit or vegetable that's been picked recently, the water is still mostly structured like we discussed in the Water chapter. Letting it sit for weeks or months in the back of a truck or a store shelf destructures the water and the water content evaporates. This means you don't get as much of the benefit.

Do you really need fiber? Dietary requirements claim you need thirty grams of fiber a day in order to have regular, comfortable bowel movements. That's a myth. The truth is that people on the carnivore diet have zero grams of fiber, and they're fine. Let's discuss fiber. There are two types of fiber: soluble and insoluble.

Soluble fiber pulls water into the gut to soften a stool. It feeds microbes in your gut, slows the absorption of sugars and may block some absorption of cholesterol. Thus, we don't get sugar spikes. Insoluble fiber, on the other hand, does not feed microbes in your gut. It creates bulk in the stool and helps trap cholesterol and excrete it out.

Okay. We are going to get gross again and talk about poop. Do you know what a majority of this stinky brown stuff is? Dead bacteria and water. This makes up approximately seventy-five percent. The rest is dead skin cells sluffed off your gastrointestinal lining, some fats, and excess cholesterol. Insoluble fiber is also present if you consume it.

The theory goes that this slowing down of digestion keeps you fuller longer and acts like a broom cleaning your gut walls. But could it also be "scraping" them, causing inflammation? There are very few studies looking at this, but logically, it makes sense. Here's another good analogy, my students.

Close your eyes and take deep breaths through your nose (of course, ha ha). Imagine you're at the waterpark with your family. As you go down the slide, the water turns off. Oops! All of a sudden, you're screeching along and your ass and back are burning due to the friction. Now, imagine that the waterslide is your digestive tract and the poop is YOU. You see a problem here? Water irrigates and cools the slide. Lack of it causes inflammation and irritation. Now do you see why you should drink lots of structured water?

Fiber in the context of a high-carb diet does have some minor benefits, though. The microbiome breaks down this fiber in your colon and turns it into fatty acids. What else is a fatty acid that we've already discussed? Butter! Now no need to freak out about your fiber consumption. Stopping or reducing dietary fiber intake reduces constipation and its associated symptoms (World Journal of Gastroenterology 2012, Sept 7; 18(33):4593-45960).

Fulvic and humic acids: We already briefly discussed this earlier in the chapter, but it's worth repeating. We're destroying the soil through monocropping and pesticides. And that means we're destroying the fulvic and humic acids created by the soil's microbes. Fulvic and humic acid are what give plants the majority of their nutrients. They convert inorganic minerals like calcium and magnesium in the soil into organic ionic minerals, which can be absorbed by the plant roots, and then by humans eating the plants. Fulvic and humic acids are probably one of the most important complexes you should be supplementing with.

You can take supplements of fulvic and humic acid to help rebalance the food you're eating. The one I take is called Vital Earth. The manufacturer mines ancient plant deposits where the vegetation is still fertile and extracts the fulvic and humic acid. This miracle molecule acts as a detoxifier, antioxidant, and nutrient enhancer, among a myriad of other benefits. When you take it, you're getting the same benefits the plant is getting. Remember, mineral deficiencies are on the red side of the model.

Salt intake: How many times have you heard that salt's bad for you? And that you need to be on a low-salt diet because salt causes hypertension, type 2 diabetes, and heart attacks? This is partially true in the context of a high-carb, processed food or SAD (standard American diet). All of this processed food is ultimately contributing to disease, just as our model shows, and consequently disrupting the natural salt balance in the body. Real unprocessed salt is essential for health. This is also demonstrated in my model under "mineral deficiencies" as salt is a mineral. Furthermore, what kind of chemically treated salt is in processed food? Iodized!

What they forget to tell you is that iodized salt has been stripped of its minerals. It's processed and refined. Anything that's processed and refined is going to cause inflammation, and that's what causes the problem, not the salt itself. It's about balance. If you aren't eating an ultra-processed diet, you're getting water content and good salt. Therefore, a *low*-natural salt diet is probably not the best choice for you. Why? Because water, minerals, and salt are essential for health. There are two "oceans" in our cells, intracellular and extracellular, and they must always be in balance. When you're eating a whole-food diet, the oceans are in balance. If you do this, everything is hunky-dory. Notice how no one really talks to us about this component.

Instead of typical refined table salt, try Himalayan, Celtic, sea, and bamboo salts that have trace minerals and are not refined. Then, you can salt your food to taste. If you're eating a proper diet with no processed foods and sugars, you're most likely eating the right amount of salt.

Remember that water needs minerals to start the nucleation process (crystallization and structuring of water around a mineral). You just have to make sure the salt is natural, not iodized.

A quick note. When shopping at supermarkets, stay around the perimeter of the store. This is where the real food is and not the "Frankenfood."

When vegans say that you need to feed the gut microbiome fiber, well, there is an alternative. It's called animal protein. But whatever eating style you choose to adopt—carnivore, keto, vegan, vegetarian, etc.—remember that a SAD (standard American diet) is not the ideal choice for longevity unless you enjoy stressful visits to the doc. I don't! As far as these outlier ways of eating go (carnivore, keto), millions of people enjoy success eating this way, me included.

Food impacts your body in a number of ways. But armed with these simple rules, you'll be able to use food to help you stay strong and healthy and let go of the adversarial relationship that ultra-processed food has with your body.

When you do that, you create healthier patterns that are ready to work for you. Next, we talk about movement and how you can use your body to stay even healthier.

WHY ARE YOU SICK?

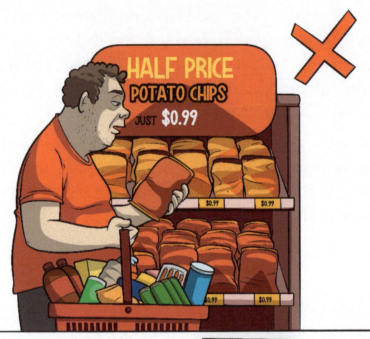

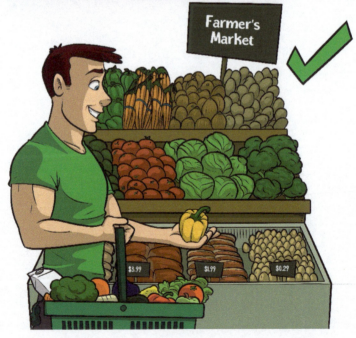

Let food be thy medicine, thy medicine shall be thy food.
~Hippocrates

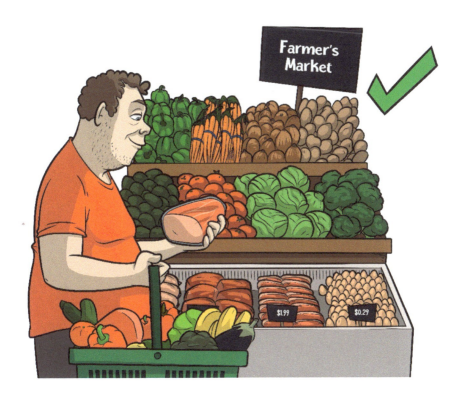

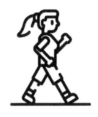

CHAPTER 8
Movement

Today I will do what others won't, so tomorrow I can accomplish what others can't.
~ Jerry Rice

I've talked about my past as a hopeful bodybuilder. I was terrified of being skinny, and I compensated by building as much muscle as possible. I ate protein powders and had six meals a day. I never missed a single meal.

With all of that exercise, you would think that I would have been in the best shape of my life. But a few months after my fortieth birthday, one of my friends poked me in the belly and laughed. "Hey Ben, you need to lose some weight there. Looks like you're getting a little fat."

I was horrified. I went and looked in the mirror,

and I saw that while the rest of my body was still slim, I was growing a gut. It looked a lot like a beer belly, a slab of fat growing despite all of that exercise.

I was working out every day: lifting weights, going to the gym, getting my heart rate up. But I wasn't drinking energized, structured water yet. I hadn't started my low-carb diet. I was sleeping with my mouth open. All of those things were causing chronic inflammation and chronic stress. I was totally unaware.

It took me years to get healthy because I was blindly following the advice that I heard all around me. "Exercise and diet are the key to losing weight." Ironically, this advice is flawed because exercise is only a small fraction of the equation (and when I say small, I mean tiny. Think approximately five percent). But I didn't use my own head and my own critical thinking skills. I did what everyone told me to do.

After just two years of giving up carbs, drinking energized, structured, mineral-rich water, and making other lifestyle changes, my gut is entirely gone. Now, my body has adapted to utilizing fat for energy and not carbs. I'm in the best shape of my life in my fifties. I can eat fifteen hundred calories a day or a thousand calories in a day and still gain muscle. Heck, I can skip meals for two days without losing muscle because I'm on a low-carb diet. I'm using the term "calories" generically. As I will discuss later, calories are an incomplete measurement of the way you lose weight.

Why, might you ask? Because my body has become metabolically flexible. I can metabolize fat, protein, or carbs for energy. When you aren't metabolically flexible, the body burns carbs first and then protein because it isn't efficient at accessing fat. When fat-burning enzymes become "up-regulated" (awakened from dormancy) from a low-carb diet, the body can utilize protein for muscle building or repair. Why would your body want to use protein for energy if it doesn't have to? Think *that* out while you scratch your head. It's the building blocks of tissue. Also, understand the body has to use carbohydrates first because, in excess, they are toxic to the cells.

That doesn't mean exercise isn't beneficial to your health. Exercise can increase brain function and reduce inflammation. One of the most important functions of exercise is that it increases mitochondrial biogenesis, meaning more mitochondria and bigger mitochondria in the cells. Light bulb moment — do you know one of the tissues that has the most mitochondria? In ye ol' muscles, damn it! Keep working out! Remember the images of the power lines in Chapter Three powering the city?

Remember, mitochondria are what produce

energy in cells. So the more of these energy factories you have in your body, the more energy you produce and the more water you can store. The more water you can store equates to helping you stay hydrated. So, lack of exercise leads to mitochondrial dysfunction, which further leads to chronic dehydration. Dehydration is the root cause of many problems (See the Water Chapter).

What all of this means is that if you want to understand why you're sick and reclaim your health, you need to completely reevaluate what the green side benefits actually are—and how to take advantage of them.

The Path to Weight Loss

Movement is important to your health in many ways. Again, it builds muscle, which holds more water than fat, allowing more structured water to be held in your system. How does it do this? Through mitochondrial biogenesis, as I mentioned. Muscle is the key to longevity. Mitochondria are *so* important they have their own circle in our model.

This super organelle inside the cells also helps to structure the water you drink. More mitochondria equals more structured water equals a probable longer life span. It gives you more energy and increases the production of chemicals that improve your mood by balancing your hormones. When you learn how to move in a way that supports a healthy body by nourishing these organelles, you will be on a path to greater health and vitality. You better make mitochondria your best friend. All you have to do is look at the model. I'm hammering home that all the factors on the green side help you and all the factors on the red side hurt you.

The other reason building muscle and maintaining muscle mass is vital for your longevity is because more muscle means more efficient metabolism. Let's get geeky again. More muscle encourages the growth of new blood vessels. This, in turn, helps nourish the cells and remove waste products more effectively. Your engine (body) keeps firing on all cylinders. Remember earlier when we talked about glycocalyx? When you damage this lining of the blood vessels through all the red lifestyle factors, you also damage the capillaries (the small blood vessels that makeup ninety-nine percent of the vasculature). The capillaries are what feed your vital organs. See a problem here? You need all those little capillaries. The more muscle you have, the more "highways" (capillaries) you have that help remove waste and deliver nutrients. Now you are more educated than many doctors on this topic!

With all of these great reasons to exercise, it's shocking that one the weight-loss industry touts is so completely accurate. The truth is, exercise *does very little to help you lose weight.*

It's a hard fact to accept, but it's true. You might lose a small amount of water weight when you first start exercising. But if you're at the gym, sweating away on the stair climber, you're not doing your body any good. Why? Just look back at the Ultimate Health Model™. The more each red circle is aggravated, the worse off you are, and the more difficult it will be to lose fat. I'm making the distinction between weight and fat deliberately, by the way. Weight is too ambiguous. Most people want to lose fat.

As an example, the more chronic inflammation a person has, the harder it is to lose fat. On the flip side, the more you utilize the green side of the Ultimate Health Model™, the easier it is. Losing fat and getting healthy is really as simple as following the positive lifestyle factors. On top of that, chronic long bouts of exercise like aerobics actually stress your entire system with an influx of cortisol, a stress hormone that hurts your body when it is out of balance.

A word of caution about marathons or triathlons. This might cause too much chronic stress on the body. Where you are on the pendulum of the model determines what you can (should) do. The ball is in your court.

Also, you can't "target" certain areas where you want to lose weight. The body uses fat wherever it deems necessary. You can pay for targeted procedures like liposuction, but that might lead to complications down the road. Plus, the body will position fat where it wants to even after a procedure if you're not eating the right diet.

Dieting also doesn't lead to long-term weight loss. Dieting stresses the body. "Calories in, calories out" is not an accurate or effective way to lose fat. This is not "new news" and is definitely debatable. Did you know that ingredient labels can be off their calorie count by as much as twenty percent up or down? That's a whopping forty percent margin for error. Also, calories are a measure of heat or energy. We don't eat heat or energy, and both have no relation to mass consumed or released.

Furthermore, calories are a very inaccurate way to measure food intake because of our model. If you're chronically dehydrated and have chronic inflammation, those calories are going to be processed differently than if you were not chronically inflamed.

We eat food that is chemically converted to energy. The problem with calorie-restricted diets is that the minute you go off the diet and start eating the processed garbage that caused the problem, your body will store everything as fat. Even a piece of lettuce! It doesn't want to be starved again. Your body is not stupid, and you can't trick it.

The whole diet and exercise industry is built on false assumptions. They tell you that it's your fault you're overweight. You have a lack of willpower. Just control yourself. Don't eat as much. They put the blame on you—and that isn't fair.

No matter how perfectly you diet, the effects will be minimal as long as you are still engaging the lifestyle factors on the red side. I believe you lose weight (fat) by reducing these factors as much as possible or practical, impacting your health. If you breathe through your nose, you lose weight. If you drink structured, mineral-rich water, you lose weight. If you eat the right diet and cut out sugar, you lose weight. It's that damn simple!

If you're overweight, starting an intense exercise regime is likely the worst thing you can do. You don't have a fat problem. You have an "imbalance in the red circles of the health wheel" problem. Chronic exercise further imbalances the circles and makes it even worse. Before you can start exercising, which is healthy for you, you have to understand and address these circles. I can't overstate enough how crucial and important these circles are in understanding your health challenges.

Don't Exercise for Abs

Exercise doesn't create muscle definition. I have a six-pack, but it isn't from sit-ups. In fact, I don't do any of that hard, directed exercise. The truth is that we all have a six-pack—it's just hidden under fat. You don't need to build muscle to develop a six-pack. You just need to balance the factors on our model to reduce fat and make your six-pack visible. Remember this simple yet powerful phrase: "Abs are built in the kitchen!"

Exercise isn't the path toward weight loss. But if exercise can't help you in that area—what *can* it do for you?

The Real Benefits of Exercise

Exercise has a huge number of benefits for your body. Besides building muscle mass—we've already discussed those benefits—it improves your brain function, it's good for balancing hormones, and it's good for blood flow. It also helps in other ways:

- Allows your body to hold more structured water
- Creates more mitochondria in a process called mitochondrial biogenesis
- Improves your lymph flow and blood flow
- Balances your hormones
- Turns all the circles on the green side for optimum health

This is the answer to your health problems. Let's look at each of these points in more detail.

In Chapter 6, you learned all about structured

water. The more structured water you have in your body, the longer you are likely to live. Remember, it takes a great deal of your body's energies and resources to structure water. Muscle holds more water than fat, so the more muscle you have, the more water you can hold. It's a simple and straightforward equation that I hope makes sense.

I'm going to say it again: muscle is one of the organs with the most mitochondria. Guess what's also a muscle? Your ticker, or heart. We already discussed how important mitochondria are earlier in the chapter, but it bears repeating. Take care of your mitochondria like they are your children. And that's a lot of children! I heard this analogy, which I thought was spot on about these powerhouses. Think of them like money. The more money you have, the more choices you have. The body currency is mitochondria. The more cellular energy from healthy, abundant mitochondria, the more choices you have!

Your lymph nodes and vessels are the waste removal system of your body. Your blood vessels transport blood, but the lymph vessels transport waste products out of the cells. Your heart beats and moves your blood, so what creates motion to move your lymph fluid? Exercise. When you move your body, you literally detoxify your cells and organ systems.

Finally, exercise is a great way to balance your hormones: testosterone, estrogen, and progesterone levels are all impacted by exercise.

There's one other hormone that exercise impacts: cortisol, your stress hormone. Let's look at stress in more depth.

The Stress Hormone

Clammy palms. Racing heart. Short breaths. No one loves to feel stress. But the fact is that you can't stay in a relaxed state all day, every day, for the rest of your life.

Short bursts of stress are actually good for you because they teach your body what to do, and it's an adaptive process. That's why short burst activities that raise your heart rate, like sprinting, burpees, or jumping rope, are good for you. But it's easy to overdo it and start hurting your body.

I bet you've never heard the term "chronic exercise" before. It's what I call long-term, sustained exercise, stretched out on a daily basis. It's not optimal for your body. It raises your cortisol levels and keeps them up for way too long. That causes chronic stress, with no chance for your body to recover, learn, and adapt to the stress.

It also keeps your heart rate in the red zone for way too long. If your heart rate is in the upper ranges (adjusted for age), it is very stressful on the body on a chronic basis. Below that range is fine. For short periods, above that upper range is fine too. That's why high-intensity interval training is good. It causes stress, but it's acute stress that causes adaptive changes in your body.

You might think that most professional athletes are in great shape, but people who exercise too much most likely have very high levels of chronic inflammation. This might explain why endurance athletes like long-distance runners might suffer from heart attacks. They think that they're in great shape, but they're putting their heart and other organs under way too much stress. Remember that we discussed where fat is stored in the body in earlier chapters? You can have metabolically problematic visceral or liver fat and still be thin. It all depends on where you stand on the model and your health status.

Jogging Is a Killer

On top of the negative stress impact of running, it's not ideal for your hips and knees. That's because most people jog and run on concrete. Concrete is not your friend. It has no give to it, unlike sand, dirt, or grass. Do you know how much pressure that puts on your joints and ligaments? If you do want to exercise by running, you need to do it in sprints, not long-haul runs, preferably on grass, sand, or dirt—and if possible, barefoot. That way, you get all the benefits of exercise, as well as the benefit of grounding (revisit

Chapter Three and burn it into your brain).

Sitting is also a slow killer. This is not debatable. You might have heard the phrase thrown around recently, "Sitting is the new smoking." This might sound far-fetched, but it's true. Prolonged periods of sitting actually decrease glucose tolerance and increase insulin resistance. This is also going to come as a shock; if you think you can just exercise your way out of sitting in your cubical for eight hours daily, that ain't gonna happen! Extended sedentary periods are independent of exercise! Think about our ancestors: they were always moving. In our modern society, our butts are glued to chairs in the name of productivity! Well, it's actually backfiring, with low back pain being one of the top reasons for hospital visits. I highly recommend a stand-up desk. Hell, you could do laps around your office if you have, too. Just move, as we talk about next.

Get Moving—Gently

Before you start on this new exercise regime, remember that ALL the factors on the green side, especially nose breathing, structured water, and proper sleep are foundational if you want to see results!

As you start exercising, try to get outside and into the sunlight. Sunlight helps your blood flow and helps to structure the water in your body. Sunlight probably prevents heart attacks and keeps inflammation down. Take the opportunity to embrace two cures in one "pill." Ironically, gyms can be a good choice if you want to weight train and do resistance exercises. Emphasis on starting slowly and moving gently. I also strongly recommend getting a trainer. My trainers are awesome. They keep me accountable, and I've seen tremendous gains. And don't think a trainer is only for the newbies in the gym. I've been working out, as you know, for the better part of forty years.

Pilates is another great way to get more fit. I used to think, *Pilates? Isn't that for sissies and new-age hippies?* Boy, was I wrong! Pilates is one of the best exercise practices to strengthen the core, ligaments, and tendons as well as tone muscles, improve flexibility, and keep you walking upright into your golden years. A shout-out to my instructor! She's awesome!

Play is exercise. Climb a tree. Play with your kids outside. Do cartwheels on the beach. Move your body and have fun.

If you're grossly overweight or obese, for that matter, I suggest you focus on the other principles in the book first in order to tackle your weight loss. But that doesn't mean you can't start moving. Here are some great exercises you can do that are gentle on your body and will provide the benefits of exercise without contributing to inflammation or the other circles on the red side.

No matter which of these activities you choose, make sure that you aren't overdoing it. It's all about balancing the excess. If you're thinking, *But I love hiking! Can I hike?* Of course, you can. Just be cognizant and aware of the intensity, duration, and type of exercise you are doing.

Gentle walking: Go for walks around your neighborhood or a jaunt along the beach. *If* you can safely take your shoes off while you walk, that's even better. You can even go on challenging hikes if that's what you enjoy. You can walk every day if you want to.

Yoga: This fantastic exercise is gentle and good for your body. Why do you think the people from India have been doing yoga for ten thousand years? When you stretch, you increase blood flow into your ligaments and nourish your tendons. Some yoga is more challenging than others.

Swimming: If you want to do some gentle laps at a pool or water aerobics, that's a great idea.

Massage: Believe it or not, I've included massage on the list of exercises you can do. Massage is all about movement—it's just another person performing the movement on you. A lot of people think of massage as a luxury, but I say it's a necessity. It gets the blood moving, and the massage therapist's touch actually helps structure the water in your body. Structuring water is the A-1 priority, period.

Sprinting: You might also be surprised to see high-intensity interval training on my list since the other exercises I recommend are all very gentle. The trick with this kind of exercise is that you create short-term, acute stress rather than long-term chronic stress. That helps your body adapt and grow, and it is great for you over time. Sprinting increases the production of a hormone called HGH (human growth hormone). I'm sure you've heard of people dropping hundreds or thousands of dollars to inject it synthetically. Sprinting is free! This is a no-brainer, people. Not to mention it doesn't have the side effects of man-made chemicals (red negative lifestyle factor) as when taking a synthetic hormone. Just make sure that you don't sprint every day. Once a week is optimal for receiving benefits. Also, understand that this exercise should not be done until you're in a reasonable state of fitness.

Run from My Gut

In 2012, when I hated my gut and was determined to get rid of it, I tried a few things before I settled on the low-carb diet. One of those things was aerobic exercise. I decided to start running every day. I told myself, *Okay, I'm going to lose weight, I'm going to get in shape, I'm going to get toned.*

There was a huge hill near where I lived, with something like a thousand-foot elevation. Every morning, I strapped on my shoes, pounded down the concrete road, and tackled that epic hill. Panting and exhausted, my hips sore, my feet aching, I pounded back down the hill to home.

I lasted one week.

I hated running. It hurt my back. It hurt my feet. I didn't lose a single pound. I was dripping with sweat and working hard, but it didn't seem to do anything for my body. After just seven days, I knew the strategy was a mistake for me.

I was doing exercise for all the wrong reasons. I wasn't using it to make myself feel healthier—I was trying to punish my body into losing weight.

After I made my lifestyle changes, my attitude toward exercise changed. Now, it's just one part of the equation that I keep in a running loop in my head at all times: How can I keep inflammation to an absolute minimum to keep my body happy?

That's not to say I'm perfect. I have some gum issues left over from when I ate carbs. I have a recurring fungus on my toes that's a sign of inflammation. But I keep it as low as I can, knowing that is the path to extending my life.

Next, we are going to discuss what probably is a main driver in the explosion of chronic disease: toxins, and especially EMFs (the radiation produced by all those devices glued to people like second appendages).

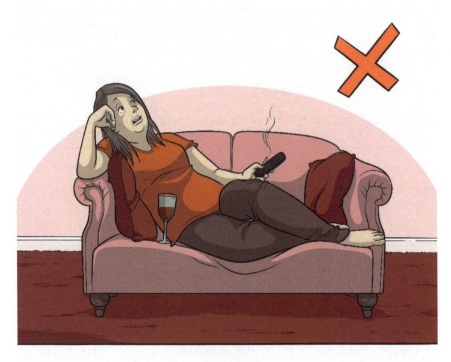

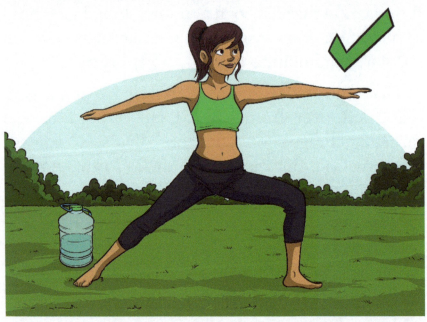

Your health account, your bank account, they're the same thing. The more you put in, the more you can take out.
~Jack Lalanne

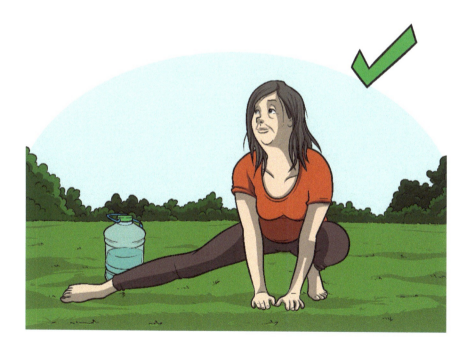

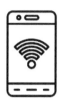

CHAPTER 9
Environment

A healthy planet and healthy people are two sides of the same coin.
~ Dr. Margaret Chan

When I was at that casino in Reno in 2022, I started to suffer from something called electromagnetic frequency (EMF) sensitivity. When you're really in touch with your body, when you're in tune with even subtle changes, you can begin to notice the impacts of EMFs on your body. Some people suffer from EMF sensitivity all the time, while other people notice the effect only when it gets really acute.

Bombarded by EMFs

Reno was the first time I had experienced this phenomenon. There I was, in a small room, surrounded by betting machines, cell phones, and even laptop computers. I felt overwhelmed. There was a pressure against my skin, and I actually felt my heart rate increase. I thought, *Damn! I'm being electrically poisoned by all this technology. If the body is a marvelous electrical machine itself, then surely these man-made frequencies are what's making my cells cry!*

It's hard to describe, but I knew right away I was being impacted by EMFs. Even holding my cell phone in my hand left me with a sour feeling.

I had to get away from it all. I was enjoying the time with my friend, but I was so relieved when we finally left Reno.

That experience caused a shift in my understanding of EMFs. I already knew they were around us all the time. But the fact that we don't notice their presence until we become overwhelmed by it doesn't mean they aren't doing any damage every minute of every day.

After my experience in Reno, I saw that I needed to do everything I could to mitigate the number of EMFs in my life. Before that, I used to talk on my cell phone all the time. Now, I never bring it up to my ear. I put it on speakerphone and put it on a counter or tabletop when I'm talking.

EMFs are just one of the environmental toxins that bombard us in our daily lives. This complex web of radiation and pollution has far-reaching consequences. But if we know what to look out for, we can begin the process of controlling and purifying our environment.

Understand Your Environment

We have been living in harmony with our environment for hundreds of thousands of years. The urbanization of our communities and our constant striving for more technology has shifted that balance. The way we live is no longer the way that nature intended. We live in a world of technology and are connected like never before. It's easy to look up information, interact with family and friends, and do business remotely thanks to the modern conveniences of power lines and 5G technology.

But everything in moderation, right? We must be aware of how to minimize exposure to EMFs and radiation while still functioning in the here and now. Think of it this way. EMFs are like sugar, seed oils, mouth breathing, and mineral deficiencies, as our model shows. They all contribute to the same thing. We are likely going to pay a major price for that imbalance somewhere down the line and we are already beginning to see the consequences.

The challenge is to minimize exposure. Go back to Chapter Three. My health model shows you how.

All the EMFs emitted by phones and computers are not inert. They're not harmless. We are already beginning to see the disease rate rising, and there's a good chance it will continue to go up exponentially in the future. We are putting too many electrical signals into the air, and without protection, that increases our risk of so many harmful side effects. EMFs are a factor in chronic dehydration, as well as all the red circles in the model. Even though limited research studies on this exist, we can deduce it from the Ultimate Health Model™.

Removing Toxins

On top of EMFs, we are constantly creating pollution in the air and microplastics in our food and water. We pollute our bodies and clean our houses with chemicals. We drink alcohol and smoke cigarettes. We have forgotten how to care for our bodies and our environment. How would you know? People are busy making a living, taking care of children, and trying to survive in a tough economy. Fortunately, a genius like me has put all this information in one place for easy access. Now you have a resource for a better lifestyle. The model is what people have been looking for.

The bottom line is that we are so far removed from Mother Earth that we need to find our way back. Toxins are literally everywhere. They're in our air, water, and food. You want to limit your exposure as best as possible. Avoid anything synthetic, from personal care products to foods you consume. Eat local, organic. One of these "toxins" is actually your devices. Again, these unnatural frequencies engage the red circles in the model diagram.

Toxins cause damage to the mitochondria. Toxins cause inflammation. The liver has to process toxins from food...but in theory, could it also have to process toxins from EMFs, too? And that's a good question—do EMFs contribute to chronic disease and the epidemic of obesity? Where are the studies on that? There are none. But you can look at the Ultimate Health Model™ and see that it's all there, in black and white.

Why should you care? Well, if you want to limit your chances of getting chronic diseases like Alzheimer's or arthritis, it's in your best interest to care. The wheel is spinning, and the toxins in your environment are a big cause of that motion.

It's easy to get discouraged and think, *I can't stop EMFs. I can't control pollution. So why should I do anything at all?* We compartmentalize these things and act like it isn't our problem.

That defeatist attitude forgets an important truth: *reduction matters*. EMFs don't *cause* cancer. They contribute to it. Pollution doesn't *cause* Alzheimer's. It increases your chances of getting it.

Think of it like a lottery... but one where the prize is death. Every ticket you buy increases your chance of sickness. Your task isn't to stop the lottery. It's to buy as *few* tickets as possible and increase your optimal health over the course of your hopefully very long life.

By now, in the book, you're hopefully ready to yell these virtues from a megaphone in front of your local supermarket. Stay calm for a couple more chapters and then you can yell and scream at the authorities who have misled you.

In this chapter, we'll be looking at four different toxins and how you can work to buy fewer tickets for each of them.

EMFs and Radiation

Chances are, most of you have heard of electromagnetic frequencies (EMFs). If you haven't, the concept is simple: every electronic device emits energy. These energy frequencies are a form of radiation, just like microwaves or energy from the sun.

Have you ever seen someone use a magnifying glass to burn a leaf? Standing in the sunlight can't do worse than give you a sunburn—but by concentrating the sun's rays, you can start a fire. EMFs are just like that. A few EMFs traveling through the air won't hurt you. But like a magnifying glass, modern technology is creating so many EMFs that they're starting to be concentrated.

There aren't a lot of studies on EMFs yet, but if

you use your common sense and put these pieces together, the picture is clear. EMFs constantly bounce from your phone to the cell tower and back, filling the air around you. They emit from your computer, from your Wi-Fi, from your smartwatch. They broadcast from your TV, from your thermostat, and even from some lightbulbs. Heck, an article on defendershield.com headlines: "Dangers of EMF Radiation Emitted by Smart Technology, Smart Homes," states that even our smart meters emit EMFs. Quoting the article: "Smart technology typically communicates via WiFi or Bluetooth, which are both forms of Radio Frequency (RF) Electromagnetic Fields (EMFs). While these EMFs are generally considered low frequency and non-ionizing, they still present health risks when we are exposed to them on a grand scale for extended periods of time.

You wouldn't take a magnifying glass, direct it at the sun, and then point it at your ear. You wouldn't stick your head in a microwave where all of those waves are concentrated. But we think nothing of surrounding ourselves with EMFs . . . all because the damage they do is less immediately visible.

That's because of how the electromagnetic spectrum works. The electromagnetic spectrum includes everything from radio waves and X-rays to visible light and infrared light. On the left side of the spectrum are the gentler forms of electromagnetic radiation: radio waves, microwaves, infrared, and visible light. On the right side of the spectrum, you find ultraviolet light, X-rays, and gamma rays (powerful ionizing radiation).

We all know how bad X-rays are for our health: ionizing radiation has the ability to penetrate atoms on an atomic level. It disrupts the nucleus and breaks it apart, which causes massive damage. But you may be wondering why microwaves are *less damaging* than visible light, according to the spectrum. After all, your microwave can burn a muffin to a crisp in a few minutes, whereas a lightbulb will only hurt you if you touch the hot glass.

Thirty years ago, we had nowhere near the concentration of EMFs that we have today. The invention of cell phones and the wireless internet has completely changed our understanding of radiation and the damage it can do.

The Impact of EMFs on Your Health

Proteins that allow the passage of ions are embedded in the membranes of your cells. These proteins are shaped like channels. Ions are charged particles that go back and forth between the membranes to help cell processes happen. Each cell has channels that use electrical signals that are designed to open and close to allow ions in. Imagine these channels as having a "voltage-gated" system. Time to pause . . . what did we talk about many chapters ago? Life is the orderly flow of electrons (electricity)! Any disruption to this orderly flow is going to cause cellular stress and inflammation.

Well, EMFs *do* disrupt these voltage-gated channels, keeping the gate open when it should be closed. That lets in too many ions. Another WTF moment and a bonus head-scratcher as well! I told you this book wasn't going to bore you like the million other repetitive health books out there!

Please understand that your body makes endogenous (internal) antioxidants to deal with this problem. The body will take care of the inflammation as long as you follow the green side as best as you can. The green part of the model mitigates a lot of unavoidable damage.

Protect Yourself from EMFs

Unless you choose to live in a cave in the wilderness, you can't eliminate EMFs from your life. What you can do is reduce your exposure. Here are some great ways to limit the EMFs that you're exposed to day to day.

Structured Water: Once again our friend, good old H2O, is here to save the day! This ordered water in your cells and body acts as a force field protecting you from this onslaught! Structured water is most likely an antioxidant.

Cell phone exposure: Keep your phone away from

your ear. I mean it. Keep it in your hand as much as possible, and don't use it at all if you can help it.

Cosmic towers: Cosmic towers absorb EMFs and convert them into less harmful frequencies. Large eight-foot towers exist for cities and neighborhoods, protecting a four-hundred-mile radius, but they cost hundreds of thousands of dollars. The good news is that you can buy smaller, personal towers to put in your house.

EMF blockers: You can find a lot of EMF-blocking devices on the market. Some scientists don't feel these devices are very effective. Do your own research before purchasing anything, and try to be informed of its benefits and drawbacks. I own EMF protective clothing with silver threads that are designed to deflect or absorb EMFs. I do recommend the clothing.

These strategies will help keep you protected and reduce the amount of harmful radiation you absorb through the course of every day.

Environmental Toxins

EMFs and radiation are just one of the four environmental lifestyle factors. Toxins are an equally important and all-pervasive factor that gets the red side spinning. Let's look at toxins in the air, water, and our food.

Air: We discussed this in the Breathing Chapter, but

it bears repeating: air pollution is a problem in our modern world. The particulates in the air from exhaust fumes and burning fossil fuels create problems for our health. Many studies show that people who live in high-pollution areas have higher rates of chronic lung problems, emphysema, bronchitis, and other diseases. We can confirm this by following the Ultimate Health Model™, but we also know that it's more complex than just air pollution equals lung problems. We know that toxins in the air might also lead to arthritis or gout or poor gut health, or even Alzheimer's. Why? Because of our model. Now it's easy to put the pieces together.

One way to protect yourself from air pollution is to breathe through your nose. This is another critical aspect of your health. Since both arms have been tattooed with our other key takeaways from this book, imprint this one on your forehead: *keep your fuc'**n mouth shut!* As you know from Chapter 4, your nose is a much better filter than your lungs. You can also try to spend time in nature away from pollution and put filters into your house to help clean the air you're breathing.

Water: We have disrespected water and filled it with toxins, microplastics, and chemicals. From my research, I believe that water has consciousness. When we pollute it, we disrupt the natural energies and structure of the water, and we energetically damage it. And if we're mostly water, we're polluting ourselves.

Reiterating from Chapter Six, you can rectify some of that damage by drinking mineral-rich, living water. You can also remember to say thank you to your water and fill it with as many positive and healing energies as possible. Do everything you can to treat your water with respect, and you will help move the wheel of optimal health on the green side.

Food: Weed killers. Pesticides. It all causes problems in the soil, and those toxins transfer to you when you eat food grown in that soil. These cause inflammation and stress, which are both red circles on the wheel of chronic disease. These chemicals are also disrupting the soil microbes, which are the basis of life. Even tilling the soil can disrupt the microbiome in the soil. We were never meant to farm at all. Think of the quadrillions of microbes in the soil as little people and the topsoil as a roof on their house. Combine harvesters (farm equipment) are like bombs being dropped on them. That's why our ancestors gathered food from trees and bushes and hunted wild animals for meat. This concept was mentioned in the food chapter, but it's so critical I want it burned into your brain stem.

Unfortunately, there's no way to completely avoid commercial foods in our modern context. Instead, we have to do what we can to find the healthiest options. Look for organic food and try to buy from small, local farms.

Man-made chemicals: You may be shocked to learn how many products in your life contain harmful chemicals. Did you know that toothpaste has triclosan in it? Triclosan is an antibacterial agent used to keep toothpaste from going bad. But the body does not like it. Studies have shown it can do everything from decreasing your levels of thyroid hormones to causing skin cancer in mice. Another common chemical is sodium lauryl sulfate (SLS). It's a foaming agent in everything from your shampoo to your conditioner to your laundry detergent. It also potentially causes endocrine disruption.

The great news is that you don't need most of these chemicals at all. I brush my teeth with coconut oil (antibacterial and antifungal), peppermint oil, and baking soda.

If you don't feel comfortable making your own products, you can buy organic versions. Just make sure to look out for toxins, parabens, and sulfates. Not everything organic is toxin-free. If you can't pronounce it, don't put it in your hair, don't put it in your mouth, and don't put it on your skin.

Guess what else is a man-made chemical? Prescription drugs. Now you understand why there are so many side effects of these drugs. It's right there on the label and on television commercials. Now, because you understand the model, you know why.

Why Does Smoking Kill?

Our last lifestyle factor is an interesting one. Everyone knows smoking is bad. But you may be surprised at both the reasons and ways that smoking hurts you.

For thousands of years, Native Americans smoked both tobacco and cannabis with no ill effect. It isn't the leaves themselves or the smoke that does so much damage. It's the toxins we put into cigarettes. Cigarettes have over seven hundred different chemicals in them, of which at least two hundred fifty are known toxins (chemicals that are directly harmful to human health). Even cigarettes with filters remove almost none of those toxins. They just create a false sense of security. Smoking causes all the red circles to be engaged at some level.

One common objection you hear from smokers is, "I've smoked all my life, and I don't have lung cancer. My father smoked for years, and he never got cancer." Well, I have a question for those people. Do you have arthritis? Do you have ulcerative colitis or Crohn's disease? Do you have type 2 diabetes? Have you ever wondered if your smoking might be causing that?

So many people suffer from chronic health conditions and have no idea where they come from—because they aren't familiar with the Ultimate Health Model™. We are, and we know that all of these conditions are connected. All of the negative lifestyle factors impact that wheel and increase the likelihood that we'll suffer from different illnesses and diseases.

The same is true on the other side of it. Some people say, "Why did I get lung cancer? I never smoked a day in my life." Well, it might be because they were overusing their phone, or eating too much sugar and seed oils, or mouth breathing, or thinking negative thoughts. And what about hearing loss? Brace yourself because this is a shocker. The accepted narrative is that hearing loss and deafness are caused by loud noises, but what if it's caused by the red wheel of doom, especially inflammation? Just another reason to follow the green side, especially if you want to hear your grandchildren someday.

Now you hopefully understand that cancer is mostly an inflammatory condition. Whatever contributes to chronic inflammation will contribute to disease. I don't like beating a dead horse, but I want to make sure this is crystal clear.

The good news is that these factors are within your ability to control. You can stop smoking and help reduce your risk. And if you're addicted, you might want to deal with it at the level of thoughts and emotions, which is our next chapter.

Respect Your Environment

I've talked about what you can do on a personal level to improve the environmental risk factors you're exposed to, but I want to take a moment to talk about our environment as a whole.

As stated in the Food Chapter, if we don't respect the soil, it's lights out. Everything around you—from the metal of your car to the wood in your walls—comes from the Earth and the soil. Every single man-made thing comes back to the Earth. If we ruin our soil, strip it of minerals, and disrespect our environment, it could mean the end of the entire human species.

We mono-crop corn and soy to make a profit, and, in doing so, kill the soil they're grown in. We need to embrace cycles in our farming, and this is where regenerative agriculture comes in. This method of raising animals respects the environment and creates a symbiotic relationship between the two. Ruminating animals like cows, buffalo, deer, sheep, and goats eat grass, feed it through the microbiome in their guts, and then replenish the soil when they defecate. It's a perfect and incredibly necessary system. And it all comes down to respecting the environment.

A note on industrial agriculture and farming. A lot of critics say that animal agriculture is ruining the environment. The problem is they don't distinguish between regenerative agriculture and industrial agriculture. One cares for and nurtures the land and animals, and the other has no regard for Mother Earth. All they care about is profits. We can't sustain our ways, and it is my belief that we will be forced back to sustainability, much to the dismay of "big agriculture."

We have to respect our environment. It's the only one we have. When the soil is healthy, the microbes actually sequester massive amounts of carbon from the air. Technology is great, but it comes at a price, and we have to open our eyes to it.

I have some good news! Thanks to regenerative agriculture pioneers like Gabe Brown of the Soil Health Academy, who owns a ranch in North Dakota, and Will Harris, who owns White Oak Pastures in Georgia, we are restoring soil health and ecological biodiversity. Look at their websites. White Oak Pastures is sequestering approximately five tons of carbon per acre from the atmosphere. Gabe Brown is working with big grain producers helping them shift their operations to more sustainable practices. Pretty cool, huh?

I know people have busy lives, but we have to take time to embrace respect. When I sit in nature or on the ground in my local park, I look at the soil. I thank it and apologize to it for the damage we are causing. It is so important, and as a society, to open our minds to it.

Our environment plays a critical role in the Ultimate Health Model™. When you understand that, you can start to make your own decisions about what in your environment is or isn't healthy for you. There are no studies saying that toothpaste increases your chances of developing arthritis. But with the Ultimate Health Model™, we understand that it absolutely can. Everything is interconnected.

You can't control what's in the air you breathe or the water from your tap. It isn't your fault that these factors impact you. But you can control how much these factors impact you. You can control your breathing by nose breathing, avoiding man-made chemicals, drinking structured water, and eating whole, unprocessed foods. When do you that, you're one step ahead. Each thing you do is a stepping-stone to help you on your journey.

Making these changes also gives you a sense of control and empowerment over your life. As you see in the next chapter, how we think and feel also has a major impact on our health.

WHY ARE YOU SICK?

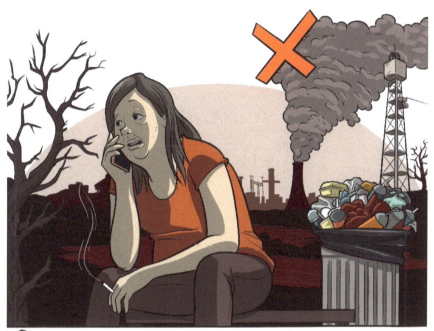

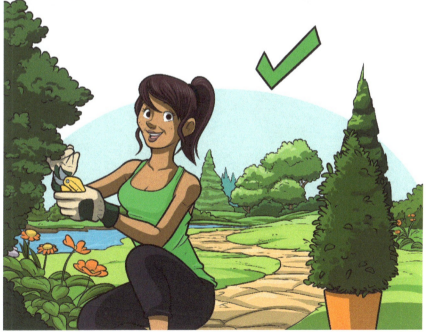

> *The earth is what we all have in common.*
> *~Wendell Berry*

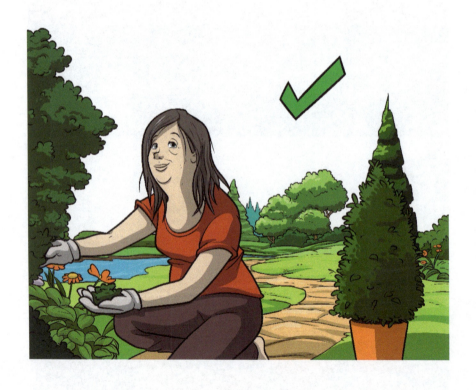

CHAPTER 10
Thoughts and Feelings

Everything is energy, and that's all there is to it. Match the frequency of the reality you want, and you cannot help but get that reality.
It can be no other way. This is not philosophy. This is physics.
~ Quote attributed to Albert Einstein, Darryl Anka, Bashar, and others

Your thoughts and emotions impact your health in a very direct way. That can be from current stress in your life, but it can also be from unresolved childhood trauma.

I experienced a lot of trauma, neglect, and child abuse from my mother. When I was fourteen, my mother told me that I was controlling the household with my negative energy and manipulative ways. She forced me to stay in my room to keep me away from the rest of the family.

For an entire year, I lived in that room. I only left to go to school and use the bathroom. My mother would bring my meals to me on a tray. I barely spoke to my siblings. Isolated, I had little to occupy my time other than my own dark thoughts.

It was a very traumatic time. I couldn't understand why she was doing what she was doing. I felt shame and grief. I thought I had to have done something to cause her anger. *What was wrong with me? What did I do?* That rejection and self-loathing permeated my entire life. For years afterward, I spent all of my time second-guessing myself.

More than the emotional consequences, it caused serious physical ramifications. I had asthma, and while there's a genetic component to that, I know that the stress of my upbringing contributed to it. I was always skinny, but I could never keep weight on after that. Stress ate away everything I put in my body.

I worked hard to clear that emotional damage. I went to therapy and learned to embrace my inner child. I fought back against the toxic thoughts and emotions that my mother instilled in me. I believe that without doing that work, I would never have been able to reclaim my health. Even if I had fixed my diet, stopped mouth breathing, and consumed structured water, all that unresolved emotional pain would have been a stumbling block in trying to implement as many positive lifestyle factors as possible.

The Western Paradigm Creates False Separation

The Western paradigm talks about the body and the brain as if they're separate, such as, "Here's what's in your body, and here's what's in your mind." It's incredibly reductionist, and we know it simply isn't the case. The mind, body, and soul are all intertwined. Thoughts and emotions *are* energy and can actually change your biology.

The Ultimate Health Model™ proves that everything is interconnected. The mind and body should be in balance. In the Water Chapter, I explained my belief that water is consciousness. Not everyone will agree, and that's okay, but I believe it to be true. And if you believe, too, then it's impossible not to see that our minds and bodies are just energy. Emotions and thoughts are as much a factor in that equation as muscles and cells.

Positive thoughts and emotions reduce stress on our cells and on the body itself. Reduced stress means improved digestion, improved cardiovascular system, reduced inflammation, increased hydration, and improved immune function. It facilitates all cellular functions to work properly.

Yes, the negative feelings you hold about yourself and your self-esteem, are stored in your cells. This is what is termed "cellular memory." Do you want another mind-blower? People who have had transplants, whether heart, liver, or other organs, sometimes report picking up personality traits of the person whose organ was donated. What? I believe my theory is correct about water consciousness.

When we start to develop chronic health problems, it's often because we are refusing to acknowledge our emotional issues. We brush them aside as if they aren't important, and then we're shocked when they contribute to our poor health.

A great way to talk about the impact of thoughts and emotions is to think of those unprocessed emotions as a form of chronic stress. We know that chronic stress is bad for your body. As I explained in earlier chapters, it triggers the fight-or-flight response, which is driven by your sympathetic nervous system. When that happens, the rest-and-digest system (also known as the parasympathetic nervous system), which controls your body's relaxation and healing, is compromised.

In our modern society, we are constantly under chronic stress. The problem with chronic stress (as opposed to situational, or short-term stress, which is adaptive) is that your body doesn't know the difference between physical stress, mental stress, and emotional stress, or what is real as opposed to perceived as real. The body is not designed to deal with this 24/7, and as a result, activates the cellular factors on the red side.

The body doesn't care if you're being chased by a bear, where the sympathetic nervous system would save your life, or if you just lost your job. The primitive instinctual response is the same: raise cortisol levels, increase blood sugars, and initiate a host of other metabolic reactions. It reacts to both situations in exactly the same way.

In the Ultimate Health Model™, stress is the major circle in the middle and one of the lifestyle factors on both the red and green sides. On the green side, you are lowering cellular oxidative stress. On the red side, cellular oxidative stress is increased. Visualize this: on the red side, it's "a vicious circle," no pun intended. On the green side, it's a merry-go-round with horsies and pleasant music. Once again, the goal is to stick to the green side as best you can.

It's hard to come to terms with that. People think, *How the hell is my being angry at my kid causing me to be dehydrated?* Now you know why. People say, "I'm doing everything else right. I eat great. I exercise. It's my husband or wife who's a pain in the ass." Well, that stress is a negative lifestyle factor. It contributes to all kinds of chronic disease. Got therapy? Therapy can be a necessity, not a luxury.

Find Your Happy

I read a study that concluded people have more heart attacks on Monday morning than any other time. The scientists who authored the study speculated that the reason for this trend is that people are so anxious about having to go to work that their hearts simply can't take it. That's why stress management is so important.

So how do you fight back against negative thoughts and emotions? You can find all kinds of ways to embrace the positive and put more happiness into your life. Let's look at a few that have worked for me.

First, and most important, I believe, is to find your *happy*. What makes you want to get out of bed? This will also help you find your purpose. It's not going to fall in your lap, though. You have to search for it. I found my happy in writing this for you, my readers. If I could put a smile on one person's face and help them on their health journey, I've done my job.

If you are stuck in a job you don't like with a boss who's an a-hole, maybe find a hobby or interest group that will help you find the happy. Maybe your children are your happy. Maybe your pets are your happy.

The Benefits of Therapy

I cannot overstate how much therapy has helped me to heal my emotional pain and stress. When you talk to someone who's an expert in dealing with childhood trauma and unresolved issues from your past, they can really show you how to look at yourself in a different way.

Embracing therapy means being open to feedback and change. I've struggled with this in the past. I haven't always listened to what my therapist has told me, or I've failed to do my homework and really incorporate change. But if you can open yourself to the process, you'll find the potential for healing is immense.

One of the really crucial things I've done with my therapist's help is connect with my inner child. When I started listening to my inner child, really being with him and taking care of him, I began to find a huge well of peace within myself.

Embrace Your Inner Child

Your inner child is inside of you all the time. A lot of people ignore their inner child, which creates all kinds of problems in their physical, emotional, mental, and even spiritual life. When your inner child is neglected, he or she will be heard, whether or not you like it, often in inappropriate ways. Your unloved child comes out in bursts of anger or sadness or grief, whatever emotions you are ignoring.

When I wasn't taking care of my inner child, he would come out and want attention. When I dated, for instance, I would be seeking validation from women, trying to make up for the fact that my mother wasn't there for me and never told me she loved me. That put huge pressure on the relationship, and often was the cause of it ending. This lack of connection to people's inner children is, I believe, the cause of most relationship failures.

Now that I'm not seeking that validation from anybody else, a lot more positive things are happening to me. I've gotten in touch with that neglected inner child and helped him to heal.

Learn to Meditate

Meditation has been around for thousands of years. What do you think people are doing when they meditate? Just sitting still and saying, "Ummm. Ummm. Ummm"? No. They're clearing their mind and reducing stress.

One great way to meditate is to visualize a pleasant place, like a beach or a mountain scene. The magical thing is that your body can't differentiate between your imagination and actually being in a calming part of nature. I hypothesize that you might even get the added benefit of the negative charge from actual grounding because you're restructuring the water in your body. This model encourages us to ask questions, and it also answers questions. And most importantly, you better love your water! Don't be shy. Tell it, "I love you, water," out loud while your friends think you're nuts.

You can try it right now. Sit with your legs and arms crossed in a quiet place in your house. Take deep breaths through your nose to relax. Some meditation techniques teach you to breathe out through your mouth, which is fine as long as you're nasal breathing most of the time.

After you've taken a few breaths, clear your mind. If something comes into your mind like, *My boss is a pain in the ass. I've got to quit,* or *What am I doing about Christmas?* don't fight it. Just let the thoughts flow through you. Look at them like a picture, like a movie screen, and keep your mind quiet.

The great part of meditation is that it works with your schedule. You can do it for one minute a day or for an hour every day—as little or as much as you want, as often or as seldom as you need. I believe the more you do it, the better you'll feel.

Adjust Your Mindset

It's easy to get angry and frustrated. Modern life gives us so many reasons for irritation. Someone cutting you off in traffic. Someone talking too loudly on their cell phone. The restaurant getting your order wrong.

The list is endless.

But when you hold on to that resentment, all you're doing is contributing to making yourself fat, overweight, and sick. You need to release those negative emotions and learn to focus on the positive. Try to find the good that comes out of annoyances, or just acknowledge them and then release them.

If you can apply some of these solutions to your own life, the positive outcome will be immediate. You will be activating the green side of the wheel of health and giving your body space to heal and rest.

It's mind-blowing how interconnected our minds and bodies truly are. Whether it's God, or the Creator, or some other force that has made us this way, it is truly remarkable. Realize that your private thoughts and emotions affect your physiology and change everything. It gives you the agency you need to take charge of those thoughts, and truly shape them for better health.

And that's something worth celebrating.

WHY ARE YOU SICK?

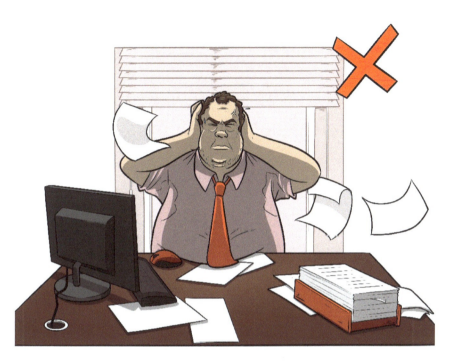

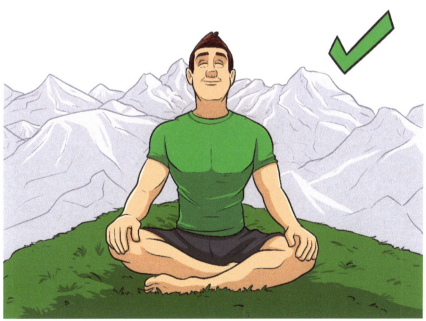

Some people cause happiness wherever they go, others whenever they go.
~unknown

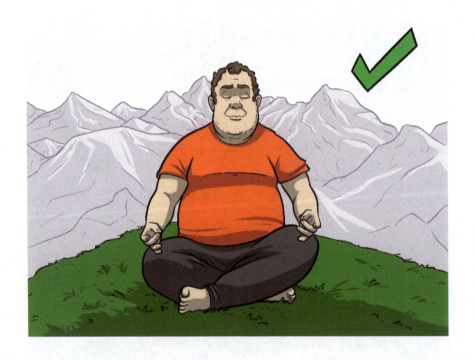

CHAPTER 11
What If?

The more you understand yourself, the healthier you are.
~ Maxime Lagacé

I told you that when my mom was diagnosed with cancer, I wanted to help. But I could only think about what I'd say to her without actually saying it out loud. "You have to stop eating chocolate," I would have said. "You need more nutrient-dense foods like animal products, and stop eating refined carbs and sugars."

I knew she would have just waved a hand dismissively. She would have said, "Who are you, my cancer doctor? I eat a lot of fruits and vegetables. Some pasta and an occasional slice of chocolate cake isn't doing me any harm." Like a lot of chocoholics, she overindulged. How awful that sugar was the drug she shot into her mouth (instead of her veins), just like an addict.

She wouldn't listen to me. I couldn't help her. I couldn't save her.

I wonder, sometimes, if she had followed the health principles laid out in this book . . . would she still be with me now?

I think that she would. And sometimes, I dream that my mother and my sister are talking to me from the other side. They're telling me that they hear me now. They see it all, and they want me to write this book. They don't want me to spend the rest of my life cleaning cars. They know I have a purpose in front of me. They're passing a message to me through God, universal spirit, consciousness, or whatever you believe, telling me this is what I'm supposed to do.

A Message of Hope

I wasn't able to help them. But if I can help you, my readers, or if I can help anyone else who will listen, then I feel like I've done my job.

This is not your standard health book. It's a whole different approach to categorical health change. It's something no one has discussed before in this context—and we can change that together.

I hope you had fun reading this. Yeah, I swore and

was a little raw at times, but hopefully, you had a chuckle here and there and weren't bored out of your mind as with other health books. I tried to talk to you as a friend and not be condescending and authoritative. I know this book is controversial, but I hope it made sense and gave you a new understanding of why you may be sick.

Share the Truth

I created the Ultimate Health Model™ to spread this message far and wide. I believe that we're going to help a lot of people. And you can help.

You have this model now. It isn't about being vegan or a carnivore or getting just the right kind of exercise in just the right amounts. It's about doing everything you can, in whatever way, to reduce those cellular players and negative lifestyle factors. Whether that's drinking structured water or breathing through your nose, or cutting sugar and refined carbs, you have to find the balance that works for you so you can reclaim your health.

It isn't your fault you're sick. But it is your responsibility to find ways to get better. This model gives you a totally different perspective on your health. I want to share this message to whoever will listen to us. And I want you to do the same.

If you listen to these things that no one has told you before, you're hopefully going to get healthy.

And then you can share your inspirational story with your friends, family, and community. Tell them what worked for you, and use your own health as proof of just what's possible for everyone.

Whether you're convinced of everything I've told you here or you think I'm crazy, I know you're thinking in a whole new way, and you're ready to try out these principles and see what they do for you. It's radical, sure, but what do you have to lose? Nothing else has worked, right?

And I'm not going to leave you in the lurch. I'm here to help you along and answer any questions you might have. You can get in contact with me or someone else from my health team on our website. Sign up for my email list, take my online health practices course, or even invite me for a speaking engagement if that will help you on your journey.

I'm here to help. Sure, I will make some money in the process, but that's not what this is about for me. I believe the medical and health establishment, in general, has let people down. I don't believe it's their fault. They are implementing what they learned in school. They are too busy to think outside the box and consequently, protocols have been stagnant for decades. Those who are fighting for change do exist, though, and they should be applauded.

You've read the book. And hopefully, you believe that there's hope. I don't care how overweight you are, or how sick you are, or how tired you are. Our natural state of health from our Creator is vitality. And now you have the tools and information you need to get back to that natural state. The journey is yours, and it begins today.

I hope you identified with the characters in the book. Maybe you visualized your own transformation with your friends through this book. If Dan & Debbie can do it, so can you! There's more to come from all of them—stay tuned! Get your pom poms, get out your megaphone, and start spreading the word.

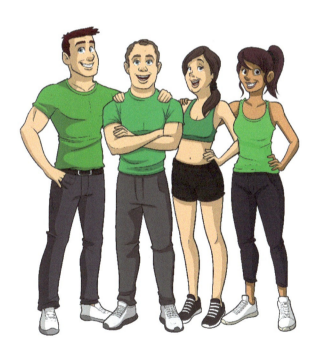

THE END

ABOUT THE AUTHOR

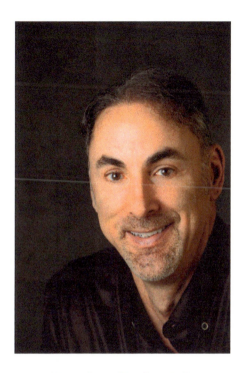

Benjamin Smith
Author and Health Coach

My interest in health started at a young age. I remember asking my dad who is a dermatologist, all kinds of abstract and philosophical questions. Why is the sky blue? Or, why does the sun cause skin issues? I was fascinated and wanted to know why.

In my early twenties I thought about pursuing a career in the medical field, specifically a naturopath. Life changed course and I got into the automotive detailing industry, owning my own company for the last thirty years.

All this time, I was still interested in health and how the human body worked but it was more of a leisurely pursuit. I read a few articles and watched a few videos here and there. It wasn't until 2012 that I became more or less obsessed with why people get chronic diseases. That year my sister died of cancer. I thought to myself, *Does the body want to kill itself?* It didn't make sense.

In 2014, I started to really dive "deep into the woods," so to speak, with my discovery of water's amazing properties. I learned water had memory and it could hold information. This blew my mind, and I started to voraciously read everything I could get my hands on about water.

Fast forward to 2019, and I realized I needed to share this information with people around me and my loved ones. I thought, *I can become a health coach!* This way I can share my information and help people get well. I signed up for The Primal Health Coach Institute after much research, as they were in line with my values. After getting my certificate, I realized I wanted to help people through teaching and lecturing.

A friend of mine suggested, "Why don't you write a book?" I thought this would be perfect. I could get my message out there for people who wanted to listen. Over the past four years, I have been researching and working on this book, and it has finally come to fruition. This "model" that I created and developed is a decade of research and reviewing hundreds of articles, as well as talking and learning from experts in their respective fields. I hope this model gives you hope and you find value in it. If I could save one person from chronic disease I have succeeded at my mission.

Printed in Poland
by Amazon Fulfillment
Poland Sp. z o.o., Wrocław